Journal of the Rosacea Research & Development Institute

Volume 1 Number 1

2010

Editor in Chief   Joanne Whitehead, PhD

Associate Editor   Brady Barrows, RRDi Founder & Director

Cover Design   Kelli Ward, in rosacea remission since 2005

Proofreaders   Victoria Albright, MA
                      Carol A. Leslie, DipCOT, OTR/L
                      Janet Roepke

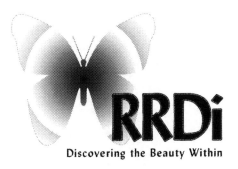

Discovering the Beauty Within

www.irosacea.org

iUniverse, Inc.
New York   Bloomington

Journal of the Rosacea Research & Development Institute
Volume 1 Number 1, 2010

iUniverse books may be ordered through booksellers or by contacting:

iUniverse
1663 Liberty Drive
Bloomington, IN 47403
www.iuniverse.com
1-800-Authors (1-800-288-4677)

ISBN: 978-1-4502-0345-6 (sc)
ISBN: 978-1-4502-0344-9 (ebk)

Printed in the United States of America

iUniverse rev. date: 02/24/2010

In memory of Karl Rebert, who volunteered to serve on our board of directors and was editing and proof reading our journal, who passed away on October 9, 2009. Karl was a wonderful young man concerned about rosacea, and had a volunteer spirit that will be missed by all of us.

Contents

Original Research

Patient Perspectives

Literature

Introduction

BRADY BARROWS

Associate Editor
director@irosacea.org

The Journal of the Rosacea Research & Development Institute [RRDi] is a periodical to be released on a regular (initially yearly) basis, published by rosacea sufferers who are volunteers that have united themselves into a non-profit organization. These volunteers have reached out to the medical community, physicians and other health care professionals experienced with rosacea along with others who have voluntarily contributed pertinent articles for us to publish.

Rosacea is a frustrating and difficult skin condition. It is confused with so many other skin conditions that mimic rosacea. In fact, there is a mystery and bewilderment surrounding rosacea that baffles not only the experts, but also those suffering with this disease. The cause of and cure for rosacea are unknown. The definition of rosacea is sometimes vague. The successful treatment of rosacea now entails a wide variety of options that sometimes become difficult for both physicians and patients to access.

Any profit made from this publication will be used for rosacea research. We hope to heighten public awareness, and that of the medical community, about rosacea. This is the first publication of its kind which has been produced solely by volunteers who suffer from rosacea. If you wish to join in our cause to find the cure for rosacea please feel free to contact us.

Most articles were contributed by the members of the RRDi Medical Advisory Consultants team. One article was provided by a corporate member of the RRDi, and two articles by members of our Board of Directors.

Editorial

JOANNE WHITEHEAD, PH.D.

Editor in Chief
joanne@irosacea.org

The Journal of the RRDi has been established to create a resource guide, annually updated, for clinicians, researchers and patients alike, describing the latest research and insight into the pathophysiology of rosacea, its treatment, and hopefully in time, its cure. This inaugural edition includes contributions by physicians, researchers, naturopaths and patients; their entries range from short insightful commentaries, to extensive reviews of the literature and original research results.

The primary feature of rosacea is redness and inflammation of the facial skin. In the first of a two part series, Dr Draelos addresses minimizing the redness of rosacea skin by careful selection of skin care products. A potential new class of topical treatments based on ophthalmic vasoconstrictors is proposed by Dr Brodell. The use of signal transduction modulators to inhibit the inflammatory response is described by Dr Stock. A common contributing factor in rosacea is *Demodex* mite infestation, which is discussed in detail in a review by Mumcuoglu and Akilov.

While addressing the cutaneous symptoms of rosacea is a necessary part of any treatment plan, many other factors contribute to the disease. Symptoms of rosacea can often be managed by modulating the diet, and this theme is explored here by a physician (Johnson), a naturopath (Kopek), a molecular biologist (Whitehead) and a rosacea patient (Cooper). As described in two review articles, stress can also be a major factor in rosacea, both biochemical (Peat) and psychological (Su and Drummond).

Understanding the underlying pathology of rosacea will be aided by considering the skin disease in the context of the whole body. Here we include discussions of the relationship of cutaneous symptoms of rosacea to ocular disease (Latkany), rheumatic autoimmunity (Christiansen), gastrointestinal disease (Whitehead) and hypochlorhydria (Cooper).

We hope that by bringing together these insightful articles about the many different aspects of rosacea and its associated pathologies, from a variety of professional and personal perspectives, we will be able to make a significant contribution to the treatment and eventual elimination of this common illness.

A New Class of Topical Medications May Soon Be Available to Treat Facial Redness

ROBERT T. BRODELL, M.D.

Professor of Internal Medicine, Dermatology Section
Master Teacher, Northeastern Ohio Universities College of Medicine, Rootstown, Ohio, USA
Associate Clinical Professor of Dermatology,
Case Western Reserve University School of Medicine, Cleveland, Ohio, USA
rtb@neoucom.edu

In the past few years there has been increasing talk of a new form of treatment for facial redness. This is a treatment that goes beyond covering up redness with cosmetics. It goes beyond current treatments such as antibiotics, which work by decreasing the infection of rosacea that aggravates redness or by direct anti-inflammatory effects. It goes beyond laser treatments that work by closing down blood vessels in the skin. This new type of facial redness drug will be a topical agent that affects the muscles around blood vessels, causing them to close down (constrict). This will decrease the blood in the skin and, therefore, redness.

For fifty years we have had topical steroid medications that have just such a "vasoconstrictive" effect. Unfortunately, the use of topical steroids for the redness of rosacea is contraindicated because of side effects. Topical steroids lower local immunity and worsen the number of and size of infected hair follicles / sebaceous glands (pimples) in acne and they can thin the skin (atrophy) and even lead to the development of stretch marks. Phenylephrine hydrochloride ophthalmic solution has been used for many years by ophthalmologists to treat red eyes by acting on the muscles around blood vessels, causing them to squeeze the red blood cells out of these vessels. You know about this drug because it is also used by the ophthalmologist to open the central part of the eye before they use their ophthalmoscope to examine the back part of the eye when you visit the eye doctor for a check-up. Is it possible that applying medication topically to the skin could reduce redness? Is it possible that this drug could be used for a period of time without losing its strength or causing side effects?

It is not time to apply eye drops to your skin quite yet. Potential side effects of drugs of this kind might include aggravation of glaucoma (pressure in the eye), blurred vision, sensitivity to light, rapid heart beat, or increased blood pressure. Whether these side effects occur may be largely related to how much of the medication is absorbed when used topically. Studies are being carried out to fully assess the risks and benefits of drugs of this type. Hopefully, within months to years more information will become available.

Ocular Rosacea: The Number One Contributor to Poor Ocular Surface Health

ROBERT LATKANY, M.D,

Physician Eyecare of NY
150 East 32nd Street Suite 102, NY, NY 10016, USA
relief@dryeyedoctor.com

I may be the first to say this, but I believe ocular rosacea is probably the number one contributor to poor ocular surface health. In other words, many people who complain of dry or allergic eyes in fact have ocular rosacea. Very often they were never told they have rosacea. I am not referring to the obvious variety of advanced rhinophyma, but of a more subtle facial redness and telangiectasia that surprisingly results in the same degree of light sensitivity, redness and irritation of the eyes. So many times when I look for the source of dry eye, I find it in facial features and history that usually points to rosacea. In dealing with how to manage these patients I focus on treating their rosacea, and usually their eye symptoms subside. Although the suggested number of Americans is approximately 14 million who suffer from rosacea, I believe this number is far greater, because the less obvious facial findings found in this more subtle group are less likely to be discovered. The patient is less likely to complain about their skin to dermatologists, but are likely to complain of eye symptoms just as much as the more severe facial rosacea patients. Therefore the ophthalmologists and optometrists are less likely to make a dermatological diagnosis, especially if it is not obvious. My advice to both eye and skin professionals and patients with eye symptoms is to beware of the possibility of having rosacea, and first seek help from an ocular surface specialist before you receive treatment to prevent an extensive workup and possible misdiagnosis. Rosacea is far more common than suggested.

I created a general health website called Medpie.com, which is a group of doctors that comment on current health news.

Rheumatic Autoimmunity as the Cause of Rosacea

LANCE CHRISTIANSEN, D.O.

lance@irosacea.org

Rosacea is commonly noted due to its obvious location: on the face! Other anatomical locations of signs of the underlying disease are also common, however, one being palmar erythema (ruddy or red palms), another plantar erythema (red soles of the feet). These phenomena, and others, are signs of an autoimmune disease caused by a common microorganism, *Streptococcus pyogenes*, the same microorganism that causes strep throat, rheumatic fever, scarlet fever and infections of other parts of the respiratory system and skin, the latter represented by erysepilas and streptococcal impetigo. It also causes puerperal fever, or child birth fever.

The inflammatory autoimmune disease manifests itself as an inflammatory vasculitis throughout the body, but certain external influences make it worse in certain locations. Sunlight, specifically the ultra-violet component, causes the vascular inflammation to be worse. Obviously, the face is "sticking out" of a person's upper garment and is exposed to the sun more than other parts of the body so it is affected more than other parts. The "V" of the neck is frequently exposed also and it frequently is somewhat ruddy and features vascular structures similar to the face: spider nevi, telangectasias, and petechiae. Often the sides of the neck are a bit red as are the back of the hands and arms if a person commonly wears short sleeved shirts. On the lateral sides of the arms, if one looks closely, one will spy signs of vasculitis with faint, erythematous, vascular markings.

Often, the redness of the face will be exacerbated in the areas of the nasolabial folds, between the eyebrows (glabella), and the ears. The former two are due to the mechanical "wrinkling" of those two areas with facial expressions. The mechanical wrinkling causes increased vascular inflammation as is noted on the palmar and plantar surfaces. The erythema on the palms is caused by the mechanical aspects of grasping, and those on the plantar surfaces due to the compression and abrasion between the foot and socks or shoes while walking.

The same variable, underlying condition causes other signs of autoimmunity and the development of various target-organ manifestations of disease: rheumatoid arthritis, scleroderma, Wegener's granulomatosis, Sjogren's syndrome, sarcoidosis, ulcerative colitis, Crohn's disease, lupus erythematosis, Hashimoto's thyroiditis, allergies and asthma, hypothyroidism, Addison's disease, Cushing's syndrome, primary sclerosing cholangitis, pancreatitis, Tourette's syndrome (which can feature obsessive-compulsive disease), and other manifestations of autoimmune cerebritis. The likelihood of the presence of these conditions is greater in patients with demonstrated rosacea.

Most physicians know the word "autoimmune", but they do not understand it and they have no idea of how autoimmune diseases affect people (and other vertebrates). Often times people get rosacea as they get older and along with it they develop graying of the hair, and it appears to be simply part of the aging process. The longer people live, the more chance they have to get Streptococcal infections and so older people are more likely to get ramifications of the disease process. Also, over time the protective immune system weakens from the effects of the inflammatory autoimmune disease, and so an aging person, perhaps, has less immunological defense against the underlying autoimmune disease.

I am retired, and no longer practicing so I do not advise people directly, only by general writing. I will say, though, that Aspirin, 325 mg, coated, three times a day, prilosec one a day, Indocin SR 75 mg (PM) and Indocin 25mg (AM), Benadryl 50 mg PM, Zyrtec 10 mg AM, Omega 3, two times a day, Penicillin 500 mg two times a day, together probably, over time will decrease vascular inflammation. The Aspirin, Indocin, and antihistamines (zyrtec and Benadryl) are anti-inflammatories; I think the Omega 3 caplets "coat" the vascular system and help decrease vascular inflammation. Since there are some indications that glucosamine helps arthritis, which is primarily caused by rheumatoid vasculitis, there is some thought that it will perhaps help rosacea, over time. The penicillin is used to decrease the frequency of Streptococcal infections, which can be very subtle and not even noticed. As an addition, use very, very thorough oral hygiene. Brush two times a day and use hydrogen peroxide, Listerine or other "germ killer" twice a day with a vengeance!

The above routine will make most people more healthy since arteriosclerosis and cancer, the two most frequent killers, have proven to be less common in those that take anti-inflammatory medications such as aspirin regularly. I suppose ibuprofen could be substituted for aspirin, but I have just used the old standard. What is good for grand-pappy is good enough for me. He developed rheumatism after having rheumatic fever three times, in the early part of the 1900s. Now we term that condition fibromyalgia.

There is no "great cure", but the above have helped some people. Heat, cold, wind, chemical irritation, in addition to sunlight, etc., will make the vascular inflammation worse. Infection, like acne, will make it worse. Acne congobata, or scarring acne, is caused by the underlying autoimmune disease wherein the local infections make healing of the lesions more slow and difficult.

How did I learn the above? By seeing 230,000 patient visits as a general practitioner, wherein I treated males and females, of all ages, for all diseases. Only in that setting could I "get a grasp" on the systemic disease, wherein rosacea is but a minor problem. The other problems appear more commonly than in the population at large, but there is a great variability in the attack-rate of all autoimmune diseases.

Inside Rosacea

BEN JOHNSON, M.D.

CEO Osmosis, LLC
30746 Bryant Drive #410, Evergreen, Colorado 80439, USA
benjohnsonmd@gmail.com

The problem with categorizing everyone with "red cheeks" under the banner of "Rosacea" is that it implies that there is one cause for the condition. Current theories have, in my opinion, been too focused on what is happening in the skin and not enough on potential internal causes. In addition, many of these theories are looking for the "Aha" discovery, when it is likely that the condition results from multiple components.

It should not be that big of a surprise that conditions involving disrupted internal physiology result in visible skin reactions. We see this with acne, lupus, melasma, psoriasis, eczema, viral rashes, etc. The "Rosacea" label describes a skin event but very little work has been done on the internal components of the condition. My belief is that all of the current evidence pointing to alterations in the skin's immune response can be explained by the mere fact that their skin is chronically inflamed and healing co-factors will fluctuate in that environment. Other skin changes, including the presence of the Demodex mite, also do not make sense when the entire picture is evaluated.

It should be clear by now that the majority of triggers known to exacerbate the symptoms are related to either events that can be explained simply (i.e. exercise worsens rosacea because it causes flushing, which makes an already flushed face look worse, etc) or they are related to digestion. Digestion is the key to this condition. Some sufferers have chronically low hydrochloric acid which results in poor food digestion that leads to inflammation of the bowel lining amongst other things. Others may have high levels of Candida which can result in an inflamed digestive lining as well. There is research on the beneficial effect of *H. pylori* treatment, which also suggests the inflammation associated with it is likely another "cause" of this condition for some. Other rosacea sufferers have Irritable Bowel Syndrome (IBS). It has been my experience that people who have IBS frequently have rosacea and have never been told of the connection.

Western medicine usually does not acknowledge the relationship between skin symptoms and the internal counterpart that is often associated with them. My approach to rosacea comes from years of watching the condition improve by using digestion-directed therapies. Some people drink aloe juice daily with positive results to help calm digestive inflammation. Others take hydrochloric acid and/or digestive enzymes with success. Antibiotics can be used on some but they will exacerbate the condition of others depending on whether or not they are dealing with Candida or *H. pylori*. Of course refraining from alcohol consumption is an obvious choice, especially if that is the primary cause of the digestive inflammation. More recently, treatments using Harmonized Water have shown promise, especially if the condition is related to IBS.

Another failure in the approach to rosacea is that current treatments do not address the specific skin issues of rosacea sufferers, which also require unique therapy. This is my area of expertise. I am not a fan of topical antibiotics, steroids or laser therapy. I believe that the vessels visible in rosacea are the result of vasodilatation and the rapidly thinning dermis (which would normally hide them). Therefore, the most important two steps in reducing the symptoms are to calm the inflammation (which will reduce the need for vasodilatation) and rebuild the dermal matrix so that the blood vessels are less visible going forward. Another problem in rosacea is that the skin's barrier is incomplete. This may be due to the rapid utilization of co-factors (from inflammation) leading to inadequate supplies for normal epidermis formation. Laser therapy collapses blood vessels, making the skin more cosmetically acceptable (temporarily) but that can result in a further thinning of the dermis by depleting available nutrients. For these reasons, the approach to the skin needs to be targeted and somewhat aggressive, but without adding trauma or further damaging the barrier of the skin. Ingredients like retinaldehyde have been shown to improve rosacea symptoms. Phosphatidylcholine is great for restoring the barrier and improving delivery of collagen stimulators and anti-inflammatories to the dermis where they are needed. Anti-inflammatories should not include topical steroids because of the tendency to further thin the skin, which will result in more visible capillaries. Wild cherry bark and willow herb (not bark) extract have shown good efficacy at calming inflamed skin. Obviously anything exfoliating should be avoided as should artificial additives and inflammatory preservatives whenever possible. So much of the sensitivity of rosacea skin is that the open barrier allows irritants in more readily.

In summary, rosacea sufferers need to evaluate their condition closely before selecting a method of treatment. Do most of their meals result in increased redness? That may mean they need hydrochloric acid and/or digestive enzymes. Is sugar a key trigger? That would suggest Candida is the culprit and many antifungal therapies can be effective. If they have symptoms of or have been diagnosed with IBS then they should consider Digestive Health (by Harmonized Water). If they drink alcohol, and that appears to be the main cause, then aloe juice will help, along with abstinence. Probiotics can also be helpful for many of these situations. As for the skin, the solutions are not easy. They need to search out the proven ingredients and consider the ramifications of collapsing blood vessels in their skin. Any tissue in the body that is in a state of smoldering inflammation (like rosacea skin) will thin and scar over time. This means the longer one waits to address the internal and skin issues, the harder recovery will be.

Optimizing Redness Reduction
Part I: Rosacea and Skin Care

ZOE DIANA DRAELOS, M.D.

zdraelos@northstate.net

Rosacea patients form a subset of the population with sensitive skin, making the selection of skin care products and cosmetics problematic. Ingredients that typically cause little difficulty in the average patient can cause severe stinging and burning in the rosacea patient. Sometimes the adverse reaction can be invisible, but more typically, it is characterized by the rapid onset of facial flushing. For this reason, developing a methodology for product recommendations in the rosacea patient becomes important. This article is part of a two part series discussing methods of optimizing redness reduction through the use of skin care products, cosmetics, and cosmeceuticals. While it is clear that prescription therapy is necessary for the reduction of inflammatory papules and pustules, as well as to reduce inflammation, the onset of facial redness can be minimized by carefully counselling patients on product selection. Part one of the series discusses a rationale for the selection of cleansers and moisturizers, while part two discusses facial cosmetics and cosmeceuticals in the rosacea patient.

Facial Cleansers

Proper skin care can enhance rosacea treatment or, in some cases, totally negate a positive effect. No skin care act is more important than cleansing. Since demodex and *P. acnes* may be contributory in some forms of rosacea, skin cleansing is the first step to restoring and maintaining a healthy biofilm. Thorough cleansing is also necessary to control the growth of *Pityrosporum* species in patients with the overlap syndrome of rosacea and seborrheic dermatitis. In short, the goals of cleansing in a rosacea patient are to remove excess sebum, environmental debris, desquamating corneocytes, unwanted organisms, and old skin care and cosmetic products while leaving the skin barrier untouched. This can be a challenge since cleansers cannot distinguish between sebum and intercellular lipids, meaning that products that clean too well may be problematic. This discussion focuses on the use of the cleansers in rosacea patients with a variety of skin needs to include oily, normal, and dry skin (Table 1).

Table 1: Cleansing Categories for Rosacea Patients

Rosacea Skin Type	Cleanser Type	Formulation
Oily skin	Soap	Long chain fatty acid alkali salts, pH 9-10
Normal skin	Syndet	Synthetic detergents, < 10% soap, pH 5.5-7
Dry skin	Lipid free cleanser	Low foaming liquids that clean without fats

Oily Skin Cleansers

Many rosacea patients with highly sebaceous skin produce abundant sebum. Even though the skin is oily, over cleansing will result in shiny, flaky skin. This is due to the barrier disruption created by removal of the intercellular lipids, causing premature corneocyte desquamation followed by the subsequent accumulation of sebum. Immediately after cleansing, the face is over dry but oily again 2-4 hours later. This is a challenging situation, since cleansing does not reduce sebum production; it only removes the sebum present at the time of cleansing. This observation accounts for the ill-founded belief of some rosacea patients that skin cleansing produces redness and increased sebum.

The most basic cleanser for oily skin is soap, created as a reaction between a fat and an alkali, resulting in a fatty acid salt with detergent properties. Soap is composed of long chain fatty acid alkali salts with a pH between 9 and 10. The high pH thoroughly removes sebum, but can also damage the intercellular lipids. For persons with extremely oily skin, this type of cleanser may be appropriate (Ivory, Procter & Gamble). Aggressive scrubbing with a washcloth or other implement should be avoided when trying to remove copious sebum, since the manipulation of the skin may provoke redness. A better solution is to wash the face twice, each time removing more sebum. Gentle massaging of the cleanser into the skin with the hands followed by lukewarm water rinsing is best. It is important to avoid exposing the face to water temperature extremes, which could provoke flushing.

Normal Skin Cleansers

There is no standard definition of normal skin; however for this discussion the term will refer to patients without oily or dry skin. Soap may remove too much sebum in this population, making syndet cleansers the preferred choice. Syndets, also known as synthetic detergents, contain less than 10% soap with an adjusted pH of 5.5-7. The neutral pH, closer to the natural pH of the skin, produces less irritation. In general, all beauty bars, mild cleansing bars, and sensitive skin bars are of the syndet variety (Oil of Olay, Procter & Gamble; Dove, Unilever; Cetaphil Bar, Galderma). The most commonly used detergent is sodium cocyl isothionate. These cleansers also possess excellent rinsability, meaning that a soap scum film is not left behind on the skin when used with water of varying hardness. This is an important property in the sensitive skin rosacea patient where the soap film might produce irritation.

For rosacea patients who are concerned about body odor and desire a "squeaky-clean" skin feel, another type of cleanser, known as a combar, is available. Combars are produced by combining an alkaline soap with a syndet to produce less aggressive sebum removal than a soap, but more aggressive sebum removal than a syndet. Most of the combars also add an antibacterial, such as triclosan, to provide odor control properties. These cleansers are commonly labelled as deodorant soaps (Dial, Dial Corporation; Irish Spring, Colgate Palmolive). For rosacea patients with abundant sebum production and difficult to control pustules, this type of cleanser may be beneficial. Triclosan is not approved as an acne ingredient in the US, but is used in Europe for this purpose. For patients with normal sebum production, the deodorant cleanser can be used once daily or once every other day to provide antibacterial effects without overly drying the face.

Dry and/or Sensitive Skin Cleansers

Many rosacea patients possess sensitive skin that must be gently cleansed due to limited sebum production. These patients are usually mature postmenopausal women. Lipid-free cleansers represent a cleansing alternative for this population. Lipid-free cleansers, which are characterized by low foam production, are liquids that clean without fats, which distinguishes them from soaps (Cetaphil Cleanser, Galderma; CeraVe, Coria; Aquanil, Person & Covey). The cleanser is applied to dry or moistened skin, rubbed to produce a slight lather, and rinsed or wiped away. These products may contain water, glycerin, cetyl alcohol, stearyl alcohol, sodium laurel sulfate, and occasionally propylene glycol. They leave behind a thin moisturizing film, but do not possess strong antibacterial properties. For this reason, lipid-free cleansers are excellent for the dry face, but are not recommended for cleansing the groin or armpits. They also are not good at removing excessive environmental dirt or sebum.

Cleansing for Cosmetic Removal

Cosmetic removal is important in the rosacea patient, especially in the eye area to prevent worsening of ocular rosacea. Many of the new polymer based mascaras can be difficult to remove with water, necessitating the use of an additional cleanser. Low foaming lipid-free cleansers, previously discussed, may be used to remove cosmetics in the rosacea patient. They can be applied dry and rubbed over the eyelids, cheeks, and lips to remove both water removable and water resistant cosmetics, followed by lukewarm water rinsing. If necessary, another cleanser can be used for additional cleaning. Many of the commercially marketed cosmetic removers contain solvents that are volatile and damaging to the intercellular lipids, thus provoking facial redness.

Another product for cosmetic removal is cleansing cream. Cleansing cream is composed of water, mineral oil, petrolatum, and waxes (Abolene, DSE Pharmaceuticals). The most common variant of cleansing cream, known as cold cream, is created by adding borax to mineral oil and beeswax (Pond's Cold Cream). These products are popular among mature women as they provide cosmetic removal and mild cleansing in one step. Even though these products are older formulations, they have withstood the test of time and should be considered for the dry complected rosacea patient in need of thorough cosmetic removal.

Cleansing Cloths and Facial Redness

Cleansing devices combine a cleanser with an implement for washing the skin. The most common cleansing device is a disposable cleansing cloth impregnated with a cleanser. The cloth is composed of polyester, rayon, cotton, and cellulose fibers, which are heated to produce a thermobond. Additional strength is imparted to the cloth by hydroentangling the fibers with high pressure jets of water, eliminating the need for adhesive binders. This creates a soft durable cloth. The cloth can be packaged dry or wet typically with a syndet cleanser. Dry cloths are wetted before use.

The amount of sebum removal produced by the cloth can be varied by the amount of cleanser, but also by the weave of the cloth. There are two types of fiber weaves used in facial cloths: open weave and closed weave. Open weave cloths possess 2-3 mm windows between adjacent fiber bundles. These cloths are used in persons with dry and/or sensitive skin to increase the softness of the cloth and decrease the cleansing surface area. Closed weave cloths, on the other hand, are designed with a much tighter weave and provide a more thorough cleansing, but also induce exfoliation. The exfoliation is intended to remove desquamating corneocytes. While this may be beneficial in some rosacea patients, it may be problematic in others. The degree of exfoliation achieved is dependent on the cloth weave, the pressure with which the cloth is stroked over the skin surface, and the length of time the cloth is applied.

Many patients with rosacea wish to exfoliate their face, as this has become a "standard" part of the modern skin care routine. The hydroxy acid and salicylic exfoliant cleansers and moisturizers may be problematic in this population due to the irritation invoked, resulting in facial redness. Individuals with sensitive skin may wish to consider using an open weave cloth gently over the face once weekly for mild exfoliation. This can improve skin texture without provoking unnecessary redness.

Moisturizing cleansing cloths are also available and may be the preferable choice in rosacea patients. The cloth is composed of two sides, which may be differently designed to deliver different benefits. The moisturizing cloths contain a cleanser on the textured side and a moisturizer on the smooth side. The cloth is activated with water and the textured side is used first to clean and gently exfoliate the skin, followed by rinsing of the cloth. The rinsed cloth is then turned over and the face is rinsed and moisturized simultaneously. This cloth technology can also be used for cosmetic removal in some patients.

A variant of the cleansing cloth is the cleansing pouch. Fusing two cleansing cloths around skin cleansing and conditioning ingredients creates the cleansing pouch. A plastic membrane is placed between two fibered cloths containing holes of various diameters to control the release of ingredients onto the skin surface. Many times the cleansing pouches contain a variety of botanicals, which may be problematic in the rosacea patient.

Cleansers to Avoid in the Rosacea Patient

Some cleansers and cleansing implements may be problematic in the rosacea patient. Products that induce aggressive exfoliation, such as abrasive scrubs, may provoke flushing. Abrasive scrubs incorporate polyethylene beads, aluminum oxide, ground fruit pits, or sodium tetraborate decahydrate granules to induce various degrees of exfoliation. The most aggressive exfoliation is produced by irregularly shaped aluminum oxide particles and ground fruit pits, which should be avoided by the rosacea patient. Milder exfoliation is produced by polyethylene beads, which possess a smooth rounded surface. The least aggressive exfoliation is produced by sodium tetraborate decahydrate granules, which soften and dissolve during use. I would favor avoiding these products and using a cleansing cloth previously discussed once weekly.

Another form of aggressive exfoliation is produced by sponges composed of nonwoven polyester fibers (Buf Puf). These sponges are too aggressive for most rosacea patients. Rosacea patients have sensitive skin that must be handled gently like a fine silk scarf. Pulling, tugging, rubbing vigorously, and strong cleansers will ruin a silk scarf immediately and are not recommended for the rosacea patient with sensitive skin. Some rosacea sufferers will scrub their face mercilessly hoping to cleanse away the inflammatory lesions and redness, when in actuality they are only worsening the barrier damage. However, barrier damage repair can be facilitated with moisturizers, the next topic for discussion.

Facial Moisturizers

Moisturizers are important to provide an environment suitable for barrier repair in the rosacea patient. Facial moisturizers are the most important cosmetic in the prevention of a facial rosacea flare. These moisturizers attempt to mimic the effect of sebum and the intercellular lipids composed of sphingolipids, free sterols, and free fatty acids. They intend to provide an environment allowing healing of the stratum corneum barrier by replacement of the corneocytes and the intercellular lipids. Yet, the moisturizing substances must not occlude the sweat ducts, or miliaria will result, must not produce irritation at the follicular ostia, or an acneiform eruption will result, and must not initiate comedone formation. Furthermore, the facial moisturizer must not produce noxious sensory stimuli, which may also provoke a rosacea flare.

Moisturizers are used to heal barrier-damaged skin by minimizing transepidermal water loss (TEWL) and creating an environment optimal for rosacea control. There are three categories of substances that can be combined to enhance the water content of the skin: occlusives, humectants, and hydrocolloids. Occlusives are oily substances that retard transepidermal water loss by placing an oil slick over the skin surface, while humectants are substances that attract water to the skin, not from the environment, unless the ambient humidity is over 70%, but rather from the inner layers of the skin. Humectants draw water from the viable dermis into the viable epidermis and then from the nonviable epidermis into the stratum corneum. Lastly, hydrocolloids are physically large substances, which cover the skin thus retarding transepidermal water loss.

The best moisturizers to prevent facial rosacea flares combine occlusive and humectant ingredients. For example, a well-formulated moisturizer might contain petrolatum, mineral oil, and dimethicone as occlusive agents. Petrolatum is the synthetic substance most like intercellular lipids, but too high a concentration will yield a sticky, greasy ointment. The aesthetics of petrolatum can be improved by adding dimethicone, also able to prevent water loss, but allowing a reduction in the petrolatum concentration and a thinner more acceptable formulation. Mineral oil is not quite as greasy as petrolatum, but still an excellent barrier repair agent, that further improves the ability of the moisturizer to spread, yielding enhanced aesthetics. The addition of glycerin to the formulation will attract water from the dermis, speeding hydration. It is through the careful combination of these ingredients that facial moisturizers can be constructed to prevent facial redness.

Some basic moisturizer recommendations for rosacea patients are listed in Tables 2 and 3. These products were selected from those routinely sampled to dermatologists, and organized by skin type. Table 2 lists moisturizers for day wear that contain sunscreen, an important ingredient for the rosacea patient, since redness is worsened by chronic UV exposure. Table 3 lists products appropriate for night time use, also arranged by skin type.

Table 2: Sunscreen-Containing Moisturizers

Name	Skin Type
Neutrogena Oil Free Moisture, SPF 15	oily
Olay Complete Defense Moisture Lotion, SPF 15	oily to normal
Neutrogena Moisture, SPF 15	normal
Purpose Moisturizer, SPF 15	normal
Cetaphil Daily Facial Moisturizer, SPF 15	normal to dry

Table 3: Moisturizers for Night Wear

Name	Skin Type
Olay Total Effects	oily to normal
Cetaphil Moisturizing Cream	normal to dry
CeraVe Moisturizing Cream	normal to dry
Olay Active Hydrating Beauty Fluid	normal to dry

Summary

The rosacea patient may pose a challenge to the dermatologist aiming to give practical advice on the selection of skin care products. This article has discussed the basic concepts for cleanser and moisturizer selection. The key to success in reducing facial redness is customizing a skin treatment regimen for each patient. Identifying skin needs and matching products to those needs will result in a satisfied patient. This discussion has provided some ideas for supplementing traditional prescription rosacea therapy with carefully selected skin care products. Part two will examine the selection of cosmetics and cosmeceuticals to reduce facial redness.

The Importance of Essential Fatty Acids for Rosacea

Laura Kopec, M.A., C.N.C

lkopec@kopecnaturals.com
www.laurakopec.com
www.kopecnaturals.com

Most Americans are nutritionally deficient. In fact, 99% of Americans are deficient in at least one major group of nutrients, the essential fatty acids.[1] Essential fatty acids are as important to our health as oxygen and water.[2] Everyone should be concerned about this deficiency, as cancer, diabetes, obesity, and chronic skin conditions such as rosacea are on the rise. Research now links a deficiency in essential fatty acids to most illnesses and diseases.[3] [4] Current research also links these kinds of deficiencies to our diet and lifestyle choices.

However, with the lack of relevant information, or sometimes too much information, combined with the overwhelming number of disease indicators, especially for rosacea, how do we become aware and make critical health decisions? Can an understanding of the importance of essential fatty acids fill in the missing gaps for rosacea sufferers and allow one to take personal action toward better health and clearer skin?

The term essential fatty acid may be foreign to most, but it is a substantial part of our nutritive makeup of fats, vitamins, and minerals. There are two main essential fatty acids. These are alpha-linolenic acid (omega 3) and linoleic acid and arachidonic acid (omega 6). These essential fatty acids are then further converted in the body into hormones called prostaglandins, such as gamma-linoleic acid (GLA), eicosapentaenoic acid (EPA), and docosahexaenoic acid (DHA). "Prostaglandins, now the subject of the most exciting and intensive research, are thought to play a role in the regulation and function of every organ and cell in the human body".[5]

Essential fatty acids and prostaglandins are responsible for a healthy brain, correct vision, healthy skin, and a healthy vascular system. They also assist the body in its ability to reduce inflammation, regulate stress, and most importantly, participate in cellular renewal.[6] [7] [8] Deficiencies in any of the essential fatty acids are linked to cancers, autoimmune diseases, inflammation, heart disease, stroke, schizophrenia, depression, diabetes, multiple sclerosis, skin conditions, migraines, obesity, and hyperactivity.[9]

There is new evidence to suggest that essential fatty acids are necessary for good health. The American Heart Association and the FDA both recommend essential fatty acid supplements for cardiovascular benefits.[10] The National Institute on Aging proposes a correlation between Alzheimer's disease and a deficiency in essential fatty acids.[11] In addition, essential fatty acids are now linked to reductions in age-related muscular degeneration, arthritis, and blindness associated with age.[12] While there is very little direct research on rosacea and essential fatty acid deficiency, one key to healthy skin is the right amount of essential fatty acids. Even as essential fatty acids gain popularity for their effectiveness in treating major diseases such as cardiovascular disease and Alzheimer's, essential fatty acids are no less significant if they can remedy skin conditions such as rosacea, eczema, and dermatitis. For anyone suffering from a skin condition, healthy skin is not a minor benefit of a major nutrient; it is everything.

Foods containing essential fatty acids should make up one-third of our entire fat intake, not the fatty acid itself but food sources containing essential fatty acids.[13] Most Americans assume they are already getting enough essential fatty acids through the amount of fat in their diet. According to Patrick Holford, founder of the Institute for Optimal Nutrition, too many Americans are consuming the wrong kind of fat and have tipped the scales by eating too much saturated fat and not enough polyunsaturated fat, which is a good source of essential fatty acids.[14] However, too many Americans are not getting the right kind of polyunsaturated fat either. What makes polyunsaturated oil right or wrong? Whether the oil is refined or not determines the quality and health benefits of the oil. Refined oil is one that is not labelled 'cold pressed unrefined' and these refined oils are polyunsaturated fats deficient in essential fatty acids. The average consumer, who is often unaware of the health risks involved in using refined oils, uses an abundance of refined oils in his or her diet. Refined oils are missing their key nutrients, essential fatty acids, and they further block alpha-linolenic acid (omega 3) and linoleic acid (omega 6) from converting to EPA, DHA, and GLA.[15]

Manufacturers began refining oils because it gave the oil a longer shelf life, and a longer shelf life translates into more profits. Refining also makes the oil lighter in color, texture, and taste and gives the appearance of being healthier. However, the highly toxic chemical solvents used in the refining process combined with excessive temperatures strip the oil of its nutrients and cause it to go bad, although chemically altered to remove the rancid taste and smell.[16] [17] When oil is unknowingly rancid, the oil causes free radical damage, which is linked to substantial nutrient depletion and cellular damage.[18] [19] In fact, free radical damage is being linked to so many different conditions that it will soon be recognized as one of the building blocks to all illness and disease.[20]

A better choice over refined oil is cold-pressed unrefined oil. Even expeller-pressed oils are not enough of an improvement over refined oils and cannot replace the nutritive value of cold-pressed unrefined oil. Cold-pressed unrefined oils such as cold-pressed unrefined sesame oil, useful for cooking, are rich in essential fatty acids and do not cause free radical damage. These oils must be used at temperatures that do not exceed 300 degrees in order to keep the nutritive profile of the oil intact. High heat can cause any oil to take on the qualities of refined oil, sending us back to where we started.

Another valuable food source is cold-pressed flax oil. Flax oil is so valuable because it contains both alpha-linolenic acid (omega 3) and linoleic acid (omega 6). Adding flax oil directly to salads, taking a flax supplement, adding a little sesame oil to food after it is cooked, and/or eating salmon at least once a week are great whole food sources of alpha-linolenic acid (omega 3) and linoleic acid (omega 6).

Another way to get more essential fatty acids into the bloodstream is to rub cold-pressed unrefined grapeseed oil on the body. The skin on the larger parts of the body, such as the arms, legs, and torso, is a valuable avenue for transferring nutrients into the bloodstream and is often a missed opportunity to increase nutritional intake. In certain underdeveloped countries, cold-pressed oils such as olive and coconut are rubbed on the body to treat nutritional deficiencies.

In addition to deficiencies in alpha-linolenic acid (omega 3) and linoleic acid (omega 6), deficiencies in prostaglandins such as GLA are on the rise. GLA is often depleted due to diet and lifestyle choices that block the conversion of alpha-linolenic acid (omega 3) and linoleic acid (omega 6) into GLA. Deficiencies in GLA are common in conditions of eczema, arthritis and multiple sclerosis and may often occur with the use of prescribed medications such as steroids. [21] GLA deficiency should be addressed through whole food supplements. The best sources of GLA are Spirulina micro-algae and evening primrose oil supplements. Evening primrose oil contains additional benefits for cell membranes and hormones and is even known for contracting blood vessels, a necessary benefit associated with skin conditions such as rosacea. Evening primrose can be difficult to digest and is best taken with food for maximum benefits.

In addition to the quality of oil ingested, the ability to digest and convert food into nutrients is fundamental to reaping the benefits of essential fatty acids. Since the typical American diet is filled with processed foods and simple carbohydrates, digestion can be slow and sluggish and nutrient assimilation can be stilted. Simply put, processed foods may keep the body from absorbing essential fatty acids. Better absorption can be acquired not only through a diet rich in whole foods, taking high-quality essential fatty acid supplements, and eliminating processed foods and simple carbohydrates, but also with a digestive enzyme. Taking a digestive enzyme with food and supplements can greatly increase the assimilation of these foods, making the most out of what is consumed.

Although essential fatty acids are a major component of our vital nutrients, research is still slow to determine how much should be taken medicinally to address each and every health condition affected by a deficiency. As a result, it is unclear exactly how much essential fatty acid is important to overcome certain skin conditions such as rosacea. The American Heart Association recommends at least 300 mg daily of omega 3 for the average consumer with up to 1000 mg daily for individuals suffering from coronary heart disease. The U.S. National Institutes of Health recommends 650 mg/d of omega 6, EPA, and DHA.[22] The elimination of refined oils and the introduction of valuable sources of essential fatty acids along with proper assimilation of these nutrients may be so crucial to improving health and a fundamental part of overcoming so many different conditions that they are worth the exploration.

A significant number of the symptoms associated with an essential fatty acid deficiency are also associated with rosacea symptoms. Could it be that rosacea is a symptom of another condition, perhaps a nutrient deficiency? Could those nutrients be the essential fatty acids? According to Dr. Surette at the Canadian Institute for Health Research, essential fatty acids will become increasingly important to our daily intake as more and more research connects the role of essential fatty acids to cellular and tissue renewal.[23] The role that essential fatty acids play in overall good health is becoming clear. Will the role of essential fatty acids as a key nutrient for rosacea become equally as clear?

Future considerations should be made to further explore the possibility of a connection between a deficiency in essential fatty acids and rosacea. In the meantime, it is important to bring awareness to a possible connection between the two, and most importantly, the connection between an essential fatty acid deficiency and overall health. If someone with rosacea suffers from similar factors associated with an essential fatty acid deficiency such as inflammation, vascular issues, hormonal issues, stress, and visionary problems, then eliminating the use of refined oils while increasing the intake of essential fatty acids may be the missing link to improving an individual's health. Furthermore, reducing the occurrence of free radical damage and consuming a key nutrient vital to preventing all disease may directly or indirectly play a key role in overcoming rosacea.

References

[1]   Sellman, S. (2008). Nature's Free Radical and Inflammation Solution. Total Health, 30(2), 46-47

[2]   Holford, P. (1999). The Optimum Nutrition Bible. London: Judy Piatkus Ltd., 45

[3]   Surette, M. (2008). The science behind dietary omega-3 fatty acids. CMAJ: Canadian Medical Association Journal, 178(2), 17

[4]   Holford, P. (1999). The Optimum Nutrition Bible. London: Judy Piatkus Ltd., 45

[5]   Pitchford, P. (2002). Healing with Whole Foods. California: North Atlantic Books., 171

[6]   Surette, M. (2008). The science behind dietary omega-3 fatty acids. CMAJ: Canadian Medical Association Journal, 178(2), 177-179

[7]   Sellman, S. (2008, March). Nature's Free Radical and Inflammation Solution. Total Health, 30(2), 46-47

[8]   Pitchford, P. (2002). Healing with Whole Foods. California: North Atlantic Books, 158-187

[9]   Pitchford, P. (2002). Healing with Whole Foods. California: North Atlantic Books, 175-176

[10]   Studies Find New Omega-3 Benefits. (2007, July). Tufts University Health & Nutrition Letter.

[11]   Ibid.

[12]   Ibid.

[13]   Holford, P. (1999). The Optimum Nutrition Bible. London: Judy Piatkus Ltd., 45.

[14]   Ibid.

[15]   Pitchford, P. (2002). Healing with Whole Foods. California: North Atlantic Books, 171-176

[16]   Holford, P. (1999). The Optimum Nutrition Bible. London: Judy Piatkus Ltd., 52

[17]   Pitchford, P. (2002). Healing with Whole Foods. California: North Atlantic Books, 179-181

[18]   Sellman, S. (2008, March). Nature's Free Radical and Inflammation Solution. Total Health, 30(2), 46-47

[19]   Ibid.

[20]   Surette, M. (2008). The science behind dietary omega-3 fatty acids. CMAJ: Canadian Medical Association Journal, 178(2), 180

[21]   Pitchford, P. (2002). Healing with Whole Foods. California: North Atlantic Books, 173-175

[22]   Studies Find New Omega-3 Benefits. (2007, July). Tufts University Health & Nutrition Letter.

[23]   Surette, M. (2008). The science behind dietary omega-3 fatty acids. CMAJ: Canadian Medical Association Journal, 178(2), 180

Food Choices for Rosacea Immunity

Laura Kopec, M.A., C.N.C

lkopec@kopecnaturals.com
www.laurakopec.com
www.kopecnaturals.com

We are exposed to thousands more toxins than previous generations and the numbers are growing. We cannot eliminate all the toxins from our lives, but we can strive to eliminate the toxins in our food. The food choices we make can be a very powerful tool to improve our health and take action against illness and disease. But it is growing more and more difficult to know exactly what food choices to make, especially with current advertising and buying trends promoting the word "natural" on foods that may contain only a small percentage of natural ingredients. Where does this leave the average consumer, especially one with rosacea?

One of the theories as to the cause of rosacea is rosacea as an immune disorder. An immune disorder is the result of a weakened immune system. One way to strengthen the immune system is by making certain food choices. If strengthening the immune system is possible through better food choices, and strengthening the immune system can improve rosacea, then making better food choices can have a profound effect toward overcoming rosacea. Therefore, the purpose of this article is to examine a sampling of foods that contribute to a weakened immune system and should be avoided, and food sources that can benefit an already healthy rosacea diet.

The most weakening food in the typical American diet is white flour. White flour, a refined version of wheat, is a staple in the American diet, but unfortunately the human body does not see white flour as a nutritional food source. As a result, the consumption of white flour in excessive amounts can eventually lead to different systems breaking down. These breakdowns can lead toward major illness and disease, including diabetes.[1]

When wheat is refined into white flour and consumed; the body has a great deal of difficulty digesting this modified grain. This modification makes bread softer and whiter, but in exchange robs the grain of most of its nutrients.[2] Quietly the body suffers from a loss of these key nutrients, nutrients responsible for making bodily systems run properly. When our bodily systems suffer, so do our organs. The skin, our largest organ, cannot help but be affected by the consumption of white flour. The connection between a skin condition and white flour is not commonly known, but the benefits are tremendous for anyone eliminating white flour and wheat even for a brief trial period of two to four weeks and replacing with other whole grains.

A beneficial whole grain for individuals with rosacea is brown rice. Brown rice contains valuable nutrients for healing and contains vitamins that are often deficient in a weakened immune system. Recently, brown rice extract is being researched for its healing affects on illness including cancer.[3] Brown rice itself should be prepared a certain way while trying to strengthen the immune system in order to keep the vital nutrients from being lost. Most grains contain a chemical called phytic acid, which can be very difficult to digest, causing gas and bloating as the body struggles with the digestion of vital nutrients. The particular way a grain is cooked can ensure maximum nutritional benefits while reducing the level of phytic acid in the grain.[4] The most common way to draw out phytic acid is to pre-soak the rice overnight covered in room temperature water and drain this water before cooking. A quicker method, simulating the pre-soak, is to pre-boil the grain for 10 minutes, drain the rice, and starting the boiling process over again with clean water and cooking the grain until soft.

Many with rosacea find the reduction and/or elimination of simple carbohydrates to be beneficial to the condition of their skin. But if improving the immune system is important, it is crucial to examine both the kind and the quality of protein consumed. Especially since reducing carbohydrate consumption causes a natural gravitation to increase animal proteins.

The word protein is automatically associated with animal protein, and animal products are not the only available protein source out there. Protein, even in small amounts, actually exists in all our vegetables and fruits. A cup of spinach, a cup of broccoli, a cup of peas even a cup of blueberries all contain protein. Another place to find protein is in a whole grain called quinoa. Quinoa is an essential protein source. Prepared like a brown rice without soaking, with two parts water to one part quinoa, this grain has a light sweet, slightly crunchy flavor and can bring a variety of meals to the table due to its versatility. Many of us hesitate to look toward our vegetables, fruits and grains as viable protein for fear that we will not get enough protein in a given day. Even though there is significant controversy on the proper amount of protein to eat every day, most experts agree that 0.37g per pound of weight, amounting to about 45 grams for the average man is adequate protein consumption.[5]

If the protein source is meat, the quality of meat is essential for getting the most nutritional value. Many meats are contaminated with growth hormones that can disrupt our hormonal levels and can accelerate the aging process. That is precisely what a growth hormone is intended to do—grow the animal faster and bigger. Certainly with rosacea, where hormonal issues are often discussed, the less hormonal interference created the better. Eating meat that is organic, range free or states on the package that it is free of growth hormones and antibiotics is essential for a healthier source of animal protein.

Dairy is another animal protein that can also be contaminated with growth hormones and antibiotics. The presence of antibiotics in our milk products means traces of antibiotics can get into our bodies. Once in our body, antibiotics can destroy the good bacteria along with the bad bacteria and over time suppress our immunity. Even dairy that is free of antibiotics and growth hormones may be a problem for some. Dairy products can be very mucus forming, can cause ear infections, sinus infections and upper respiratory problems, and can be the source of hidden allergies in children.[6] Childhood allergies can often be overlooked leading to other health problems later in life. Since mucus can be a breeding ground for bacteria and germs, it stands to reason while improving the immune system, mucus forming foods should be avoided. Food such as ice cream that contains more than one culprit, such as milk and sugar, should be avoided at all cost. In fact all foods containing sugar and sweeteners can pose serious health consequences.

Sugar and other sweeteners are immune suppressors pure and simple. What was once thought of as a simple pleasure, sugar is now being examined for its role in a host of illnesses and diseases.[7] Sugar has contaminated almost of all of our processed food and is slowly destroying the health of everyone that consumes this seemingly harmless toxin. Sugar comes in many forms, and should be avoided while clearing the skin and improving the immune system. Commonly known sugars are white sugar, sucrose, brown sugar, high fructose corn syrup, corn syrup, fructose, glucose, honey, maltodextrin, and maple syrup. Sweeteners, which can be toxic chemical additives, such as aspartame, Splenda, dextrose, Equal, NutraSweet, saccharin, manitol, sorbitol and xylose are also found in processed foods.[8] These sugars and sweeteners are common ingredients in the typical American diet with the average person consuming as much as five pounds of chemicals every year, and fifty pounds or more in hidden sugars.[9]

Processed food may some day be linked to every known illness. Aside from all the chemical toxic ingredients in processed foods, the very nature of processed food confuses the body. The body was designed to break down and digest whole food. Whole food is food in its original form. Whole food has not been altered or broken down. When we process and package food we begin to mix and match so many ingredients that the body cannot truly break down all the ingredients and suddenly the body is burdened with a lengthy digestion. Energy levels can be low and a lack of good sleep is common because the body can still be digesting food while sleeping. Diets rich in processed foods, including white flour products and white sugar products can cause poor health in the heart, arteries, bones, intestines, kidneys and other organs.[10] In order to truly improve the immune system a diet rich in whole foods is necessary along with the elimination of processed food.

Even whole food supplements possess more benefits over a processed supplement. When a supplement has been derived from a whole food, it is more easily digested and more easily used by the body. One of the most important whole food supplements to consider while improving the immune system is Green Food Supplements. Green foods such as aloe vera (as a drinkable juice), Spirulina, chlorella and blue green algae are rich in nutrients and are easily digested. These green foods contain protein, beta-carotene, chlorophyll, omega 3 and other essential fatty acids. Chlorophyll, alone, is essential for the elimination of bacterial growth in the body, the reduction of inflammation which can include skin inflammations and the renewal of tissue and other important cellular development.[11] Because each green food is different each one provides different benefits for different people. It may take some experimenting with different ones to get the best results. While there is no medical proof on the medicinal value of green food supplements, green foods are gaining more and more popularity. One reason is the newly popular GLA, an essential fatty acid synthesized in the body from linoleic acid, contained in most green foods.

Essential fatty acids are crucial to overall immunity. The total benefits of essential fatty acids include brain function, vascular function, stress management, healthy skin and tissue renewal. Essential fatty acids such as omega 3, 6 and the essential fatty acid converted into GLA are slowly being recognized as some of the key nutrients for maintaining optimal health in all areas of the body.[12] Essential fatty acids can be found in whole food supplements such as cold flax oil and evening primrose oil. As with any supplement, check with your healthcare provider, especially if you are pregnant or nursing, and read the label for specifications and for risk factors.

In conclusion, the most important foods to eliminate while overcoming rosacea and strengthening the immune system are white flour products, cow's milk, sugar and sweeteners, and processed foods. Additional food considerations for rosacea are the inclusion of brown rice, quinoa, hormone free meat, aloe vera juice, green food supplements, essential fatty acid supplements and other whole food supplements added to a diet rich in whole foods. Improving the immune system can happen in stages or through a complete lifestyle change. Either way or somewhere in the middle a healthier immune system is a healthier body and can create a less hospitable environment for any illness or disease. Buying better quality meat, foregoing the bread and pasta, passing on the ice cream, can all be better choices for rosacea and for greater health and wellness.

References

[1] Pitchford, P. (2002). *Healing with Whole Foods*. California: North Atlantic Books, p. 27

[2] Pitchford, P. (2002). *Healing with Whole Foods*. California: North Atlantic Books, p. 648 and Ballentine, R. (1978). *Diet and Nutrition*. Pennsylvania: Himalayan International Institute, p. 73

[3] Pitchford, P. (2002). *Healing with Whole Foods*. California: North Atlantic Books, p. 15

[4] Pitchford, P. (2002). *Healing with Whole Foods*. California: North Atlantic Books, p.15, 16, 29

[5] Ballentine, R. (1978). *Diet and Nutrition*. Pennsylvania: Himalayan International Institute, p. 148-149

[6] Pitchford, P. (2002). *Healing with Whole Foods*. California: North Atlantic Books, p. 149, and Townsley, C. (1996). *Kid Smart: Raising a Healthy Child*. Colorado: Lifestyle for Health Publishing, p. 50

[7] Duffy, D. (1975). *Sugar Blues*. New York: Grand Central Publishing, p. 42

[8] Townsley, C. (1996). *Kid Smart: Raising a Healthy Child*. Colorado: Lifestyle for Health Publishing, p. 48-49

[9] Duffy, D. (1975). *Sugar Blues*. New York: Grand Central Publishing, p. 175

[10] Pitchford, P. (2002). *Healing with Whole Foods*. California: North Atlantic Books, p.648

[11] Pitchford, P. (2002). *Healing with Whole Foods*. California: North Atlantic Books, p.233

[12] Pitchford, P. (2002). *Healing with Whole Foods*. California: North Atlantic Books, p.171

Rosacea, Inflammation, and Aging: The Inefficiency of Stress

RAYMOND PEAT, PH.D.

Coeneo, Michoacan, Mexico
www.raypeat.com
raypeat@efn.org

> *Editor's Choice*
> In describing the pathophysiology of rosacea, Dr Peat makes the remarkable observation that rosacea has the potential to act as a model system for the study of other diseases which share the processes of neovascularization and fibrosis. This insight should promote a renewed interest in rosacea research, which in turn has the potential to advance our understanding of debilitating chronic illnesses such as diabetes, kidney disease and cancer.

Rosacea, or acne rosacea, has been defined as "vascular and follicular dilation involving the nose and contiguous portions of the cheeks . . ." that may involve persistent erythema with hyperplasia of sebaceous glands. Stedman's Medical Dictionary 23rd edition.

Light-skinned people, especially women between the ages of 30 and 50, sometimes develop a persistent redness of their cheeks and nose. It may begin as a tendency to flush excessively, but the blood vessels can become chronically dilated. Similar processes occur in dark-skinned people less frequently. The eyes are sometimes involved, with redness of the exposed areas (conjuctival hyperemia). New blood vessels develop in the area, and the flow of blood through the affected tissue is greatly increased. The tissues become thickened and fibrotic, with the multiplication of fibroblasts and the increased deposition of collagen. The cornea normally receives its oxygen from the air, and its nutrients from the aqueous humor. As rosacea of the eye develops, the blood vessels surrounding the cornea become increasingly visible, and, especially on the inner (nasal) side of the eye, the vessels tend to enlarge and become tortuous. Rhinophyma, or potato nose, has been described as a late development of rosacea.

Too often, the medical reaction is to give the condition a name, and to distinguish its variants as if they were different problems, and then to use the most direct means to eliminate the problem they have defined. A typical attitude is that "Rosacea is an enigmatic disease with multiple exacerbations and remissions, and, unfortunately, treatment is directed toward symptomatic control rather than cure" (Randleman).

Lasers or other radiation, caustic chemical abrasion, surgical planing and dermal shaves, and other forms of surgery may be used to destroy the superficial blood vessels, and to reduce the enlarged nose or other irregularities. A few decades ago, when rosacea was believed to be the result of a local infection, antibiotics were used to treat it, and some of them, including tetracycline, helped. It was discovered that some antibiotics have anti-inflammatory actions, apart from their germicidal effects, and now it is very common to prescribe the chronic use of tetracycline to suppress symptoms.

Rosacea, and the fibrotic changes associated with it (pingueculae and pterygia in the eyes, rhinophyma of the nose, etc.), are much more than "cosmetic" issues, involving the skin and eye surface. If the invasive proliferation of blood vessels can be prevented, it is important to do that, because, for example, pannus / neovascularization of the cornea can seriously impair vision. Possibly the strangest thing about the relationship of the medical profession to rosacea is that its essential features, invasive neovascularization and fibrotic growth, are of great interest when they occur elsewhere, and many physiological processes are known to regulate the growth of blood vessels and fibroblasts, but nearly all the attention given to rosacea and rhinophyma concerns control of symptoms for cosmetic effect. Rosacea is a physiological problem that deserves consideration in the light of all that is known about physiology and developmental biology.

The increased incidence of rosacea after the age of 30, and the fact that it occurs most commonly in the areas that are most exposed to sunlight (bald men sometimes develop it on the top of the head), indicate that aging and irritation are essential causes. Stress, irritation (such as produced by ultraviolet or ionizing radiation or free radicals), and aging are known to cause disorganized growth of fibrous and vascular tissues in various parts of the body. The occurrence of these processes at the surface, where the changes can be observed immediately, and without invasive procedures, should have aroused wide interest among those who study kidney disease, diabetes, and other degenerative diseases in which fibrosis and neovascularization play important roles.

A localized stress or irritation at first produces vasodilation that increases the delivery of blood to the tissues, allowing them to compensate for the stress by producing more energy. Some of the agents that produce vasodilation also reduce oxygen consumption (nitric oxide, for example), helping to restore a normal oxygen tension to the tissue. Hypoxia itself (produced by factors other than irritation) can induce vasodilation, and if prolonged sufficiently, tends to produce neovascularization and fibrosis.

Sensitivity to the harmful effects of light can be increased by some drugs and by excess porphyrins produced in the body (and by the porphyrin precursor, delta-amino levulinic acid), leading to rosacea, so those factors should be considered, but too often alcohol (which can cause porphyrin to increase) is blamed for rosacea and rhinophyma, without justification. There are many ways in which poor health can increase light sensitivity. Some types of excitation produced by metabolites (or by the failure of inhibitory metabolites) can produce vasodilation, involving the release of nitric oxide (Cardenas, et al., 2000), setting off a series of potentially pathological reactions, including fibrosis. The nitric oxide increases glycolysis while lowering energy production. The excitatory metabolite glutamate, and nitric oxide, are both inhibited by aspirin (Moro, et al., 2000).

When blood flow in skin affected by rosacea was measured, circulation was 3 or 4 times higher than normal (Sibenge & Gawkrodger, 1992), and oxygen tension may be increased. An inability to extract oxygen from the blood, or to use it to produce energy, will produce the same hyperemia that would be produced by a lack of oxygen. These measurements suggest that mitochondrial defects would be the best place to look for a general cause of rosacea. When mitochondria are damaged, active cells produce increased amounts of lactic acid, even in the presence of adequate oxygen. Otto Warburg identified this kind of metabolism, aerobic glycolysis, as an essential feature of cancer, and showed that it could be produced by stress, ionizing radiation, carcinogenic toxins, and even by a simple oxygen deficiency. Other investigators around the same time showed that lactic acid produces vasodilation (for example, in the cornea), and more recently it has been shown to promote the development of fibrosis, and it has been called a "phlogogen," a promoter of inflammation.

Riboflavin, vitamin B2, is an essential component of the mitochondrial respiratory enzymes, and it is very easily destroyed by light (blue light and especially ultraviolet). When it is excited by high energy light, it can spread the damage to other components of the mitochondria, including the cytochromes and the polyunsaturated fatty acids. The other B vitamins are affected when riboflavin's actions are disturbed.

Vitamin K is also extremely light sensitive, and it interacts closely with coenzyme Q in regulating mitochondrial metabolism. For example, mitochondrial Complex-I, NADH-ubiquinone reductase, is probably the most easily damaged part of the mitochondrion, and it is protected by vitamin K. Vitamin E, coenzyme Q, and the polyunsaturated fatty acids are also light sensitive, and they are more susceptible to free radical damage when vitamin K is deficient.

Niacinamide, one of the B vitamins, provides energy to this mitochondrial system. Under stress and strong excitation, cells waste niacinamide-NADH, but niacinamide itself has a sedative anti-excitatory effect, and some of its actions resemble a hormone. Estrogen tends to interfere with the formation of niacin from tryptophan. Tryptophan, rather than forming the sedative niacin (pyridine carboxylic acid), can be directed toward formation of the excitatory quinolinic acid (pyridine dicarboxylic acid) by polyunsaturated fatty acids. Excitation must be in balance with a cell's energetic resources, and niacinamide can play multiple protective roles, decreasing excitation, increasing energy production, and stabilizing repair systems. The state of excitation and type of energy metabolism are crucial factors in governing cell functions and survival.

The polyunsaturated fatty acids, besides their interactions with estrogen and tryptophan metabolism, promote excitation and decrease energy production in several other ways. For example, they increase the excitatory effects of the glutamate pathways (Yu, et al., 1986; Nishikawa, 1994), and their breakdown products inhibit mitochondrial respiration (Humphries, et al., 1998; Picklo, et al., 1999; Lovell, et al., 2000).

The excess excitation that produces nitric oxide and lactic acid lowers the energy production of vascular cells, possibly enough to lower their contractile ability (Geng, et al., 1992), causing vasodilation. When flushing is caused by a mismatch between energy supply and energy demand, caffeine can decrease the vasodilation (Eikvar & Kirkebøen, 1998), but when vasodilation is caused more physiologically by carbon dioxide, caffeine does not have that effect (Meno, et al., 2005). In a study in which drinking hot water or coffee was compared with drinking room-temperature coffee or caffeine, it was found that the hot liquids caused flushing, but cool coffee and caffeine did not. Caffeine increases cells' energy efficiency, and by opposing the effects of adenosine (secreted by cells that are stressed and energy-depleted), it can inhibit vasodilation, angioneogenesis (Merighi, et al., 2007; Ryzhov, et al., 2007), and fibrosis (Chan, et al., 2006).

One nearly ubiquitous source of inappropriate excitation and energy depletion is the endotoxin, bacterial lipopolysaccharides absorbed from the intestine (Wang and White, 1999). That this ubiquitous toxin has a role in rosacea is suggested by the observation that intestinal stimulation, to speed transit through the bowel, immediately relieved symptoms (Kendall, 2002). Increased cortisol (Simon, et al., 1998) and sepsis (Levy, 2007) interfere with mitochondrial energy production.

Simple nervous blushing or flushing is usually considered harmless, and when a person is overheated, the reddening of the skin has the function of facilitating heat loss, to restore a normal temperature. But even nerve-regulated flushing can involve a distinct interference with mitochondrial respiration, and can stimulate the overgrowth of blood vessels.

Cancer's respiratory defect that Warburg identified, fermentation with lactic acid production even in the presence of adequate oxygen, was the result of some kind of injury to the mitochondria. He showed that one of the injuries that could produce aerobic glycolysis was a deficiency of riboflavin. He observed that tumors generally were anoxic, and that cancers typically appeared in the midst of tissue that was atrophying, and suggested that the cancer cells' survival was favored by their ability to live without oxygen. This may be relevant to the observations of many surgeons of a small cancer embedded in the fibrous tissue of large rhinophymas that have been removed.

The relatively high incidence of rosacea among women (some studies indicate that it may be three times as common in women as in men) is not likely to be the result of greater sun exposure, so it is reasonable to look for hormonal causes. In old age, it is well recognized that men's estrogen level rises. But the estrogen industry has convinced women that their estrogen declines as they get older. It is common knowledge that aging rodents often go into "persistent estrus," and that their estrogen levels generally increase with age (Parkening, et al., 1978; Anisimov and Okulov, 1981). Several studies in women have shown that serum estrogen levels rise from the teens into the forties (Musey, et al., 1987; Wilshire, et al., 1995; Santoro, et al., 1996). Other studies show that serum and tissue estrogen concentrations are not concordant, and that some tissues may contain several times as much estrogen as the serum (Jefcoate, et al., 2001). Local irritation increases tissue estrogen content. The anti-estrogens, especially progesterone, begin declining in the thirties, so that the rising estrogen has more effect on the tissues during those years. These are the years in which the incidence of rosacea rises suddenly. Rosacea develops later on average in men, whose estrogen levels rise significantly at later ages.

Estrogen's most immediate effect on cells is to alter their oxidative metabolism. It promotes the formation of lactic acid. In the long run, it increases the nutritional requirements for the B vitamins, as well as for other vitamins. It also increases the formation of aminolevulinic acid, a precursor of porphyrin, and increases the risk of excess porphyrin increasing light sensitivity. Both aminolevulinic acid and excess porphyrins are toxic to mitochondria, apart from their photosensitizing actions. Nitric oxide, glutamate, and cortisol all tend to be increased by estrogen.

Veins and capillaries are highly sensitive to estrogen, and women are more likely than men to have varicose veins, spider veins, leaky capillaries, and other vascular problems besides rosacea. Estrogen can promote angioneogenesis by a variety of mechanisms, including nitric oxide (Johnson, et al., 2006). "Estrogens potentiate corticosteroid effects on the skin such as striae, telangiectasiae, and rosacea dermatitis" (Zaun, 1981). Early forms of oral contraceptives, high in estrogen, were found to increase acne rosacea more than three-fold (Prenen & Ledoux-Corbusier, 1971).

Lactic acid, produced under the influence of estrogen, nitric oxide, or other problems of energy formation, besides causing vasodilation, also stimulates the growth of fibroblasts. Oxygen deprivation, or damage to mitochondria, will increase lactic acid formation, and so it will immediately cause vasodilation, and if the problem is prolonged, new blood vessels will grow, and fibrous connective tissue will increase. Estrogen stimulates collagen synthesis, and it has been associated with a variety of inflammatory and fibrotic conditions (for example, Cutolo, et al., 2003. Payne, et al., 2006, suggest the use of the anti-estrogen, tamoxifen, to treat rhinophyma).

The cornea normally contains more riboflavin even than the retina, which has a much higher rate of metabolism. When the cornea is not able to get enough oxygen from the air for its needs (and if riboflavin is deficient, its need for oxygen is increased), surrounding blood vessels at first dilate in response to the diffusing lactic acid, to increase the blood supply to the edges of the cornea. If the problem is prolonged, the conjuctiva becomes chronically blood-shot, hyperemic, and larger more visible blood vessels grow, surrounding the cornea, or even invading the cornea. Many people, especially women, experienced problems of this sort from wearing contact lenses, especially when the lenses were made of materials very impermeable to oxygen (Dumbleton, et al., 2006).

Sunlight and mechanical obstruction of the cornea produce very localized effects, but those local effects are more likely to be harmful when there is a systemic nutritional deficiency or excess of estrogen. When the systemic problem is very severe, the cheeks, nose, and eyes might not be the first tissues to experience a functional disturbance. The mitochondrial inhibition produced by the action of the parasympathetic nervous system (occurring in simple blushing) can occur wherever those nerves act, and blood vessels in all parts of the body are responsive to the acetylcholine secreted by those nerves.

Sleep typically involves a shift of dominance in the autonomic nervous system toward the parasympathetic nerves, with vasodilation. Nosebleeds, especially in children, commonly occur during sleep (Jarjour & Jarjour, 2005: high incidence in sleep, and association with migraine). A 3 year-old child who had been having an average of three nosebleeds every day, during a nap and at night, for several months, also had an extreme behavior problem. He became angry and sometimes violent when he went a little longer than normal between meals. After an oral dose of about ten milligrams of riboflavin, he was able to sleep without having another recurrence of the nosebleeds, and his tantrums became rare. Apparently, the nerve-regulated vasodilation produced by sleep, combined with a riboflavin deficiency, had been enough to produce nosebleeds. The energy deficit resulting from a systemic riboflavin deficiency had probably been causing him to be abnormally sensitive to glycogen depletion, producing sudden anger. In another individual, the energy problem might have taken the form of a memory problem, or of a hemorrhage in the brain or other essential organ.

A 37 year old slightly alcoholic man with a bright red nose and cheeks was an amateur fiction writer, but he was having trouble with his memory for words, and for everyday events. Even conversationally, he had to struggle for relatively familiar words. On the suggestion that riboflavin might help his memory, by allowing his brain cells to use oxygen more efficiently, he had his doctor give him an intravenous injection of B vitamins. When I saw him the next day, his conversation was perfectly fluent, and he obviously had easy access to a good vocabulary. Just as noticeable was the normal color of his nose and cheeks. For a week, he had a daily injection of the B vitamins, and his nose color and vocabulary stayed normal. But on the weekend, after not having the shots for two days, his nose and cheeks were again maraschino cherry red, and his speech was halting, as he struggled for words. He forgot the whole episode, and neglected to return to the doctor for more of the vitamin injections. Ten years later, he had developed a medium-sized potato nose, and had his heart valves replaced. His vitamin requirements were apparently abnormally high. At first, the problems resulting from damaged mitochondria seem mostly functional (flushing, mood, memory problems, etc.) and variable, but chronically disturbed functions lead to structural, anatomical changes, as prolonged stimulation alters tissue maintenance and growth.

Abram Hoffer, who had been treating schizophrenia and senile dementia with niacin, accidentally discovered that it cured his bleeding gums. That led to its use to treat heart disease. The "orthomolecular" ideas of Hoffer and Linus Pauling were developed in a context of biochemistry governed by genetics and molecular biology, in which the goal was to provide a chemical that was lacking because of a genetic defect in metabolism. Their idea of using nutrients as drugs has led to many unphysiological practices, in which an isolated nutrient is supposed to have a drug-like action, and if in isolation it does not act like a drug, then it should be used only according to the normal genetically determined nutritional requirement. But in reality, nutritional requirements are strongly influenced by history and present circumstances. For example, when corneal mitochondria have been damaged by riboflavin deficiency, they have been found to subsequently require more than the normal amount of the vitamin to function properly. In addition, the presence of a certain amount of one nutrient often increases or decreases the amount of other nutrients needed.

When the interactions among energy expenditure and energy production, and cellular activation and cellular inhibition, are taken into account, then it is clear that any particular problem is likely to have many causes and many factors that could contribute to a cure. Lactate, glutamate, ammonium, nitric oxide, quinolinate, estrogen, histamine, aminolevulinate, porphyrin, ultraviolet light, polyunsaturated fatty acids and endotoxin contribute to excitatory and excitotoxic processes, vasodilation, angioneogenesis, and fibrosis. Carbon dioxide, glycine, GABA, saturated fatty acids (for example, Nanji, et al., 1997), vitamin K, coenzyme Q10, niacinamide, magnesium, red light, thyroid hormone, progesterone, testosterone, and pregnenolone are factors that can be increased to protect against inappropriate cellular excitation. All of the nutritional factors that participate in mitochondrial respiration contribute to maintaining a balance between excessive excitation and protective inhibition. Riboflavin, coenzyme Q10, vitamin K, niacinamide, thiamine, and selenium are the nutrients that most directly relate to mitochondrial energy production. Coffee is often avoided by people with rosacea, but it is a very good source of niacin and magnesium, and caffeine has some of the same cell-protective functions as niacinamide.

People suffering from rosacea have been found to be more likely than average to have suffered from styes in childhood, to have varicose veins and spider veins, and to suffer from migraines and depression. Hypothyroidism has been identified as a factor in all of those. Good thyroid function is necessary for resistance to bacterial infection, for regulation of blood sugar, neurotransmitters, and hormones related to mood, and for the formation of progesterone. Progesterone regulates smooth muscle tone, including the walls of veins, so that a deficiency allows veins to enlarge. It also prevents overgrowth of fibrotic tissue, and in some contexts may inhibit angioneogenesis.

GABA itself tends to raise body temperature (Ishiwata, et al., 2005) by controlling vasodilation, and the factors such as progesterone which protect mitochondrial energy production are also thermogenic, supporting the GABA system. Flushing, both by directly causing heat loss and by reducing mitochondrial energy production, tends to lower body temperature.

The sun-damaged areas in rosacea can be directly provided with some of the protective factors by applying them topically. In the same way that topical lactate can cause vasodilation and disturbed energy metabolism (Rendl, et al., 2001), topical niacinamide, progesterone, vitamin K, and coenzyme Q10 can improve the metabolism and function of the local tissues. Riboflavin can probably be useful when applied topically, but because of its extreme sensitivity to light, it should usually be used only internally, unless the treated skin is covered to prevent exposure to light. Topically applied caffeine, even after sun exposure, can reduce local tissue damage (Koo, et al., 2007). Aspirin and saturated fats can also be protective when applied topically.

Some of the benefit from antibiotics probably results from the reduced endotoxin stress when intestinal bacteria are suppressed. However, antibiotics can kill the intestinal bacteria that produce vitamin K, so it is important to include that in the diet when antibiotics are used. Some fibers, such as raw carrots, that are effective for lowering endotoxin absorption also contain natural antibiotics, so regular use of carrots should be balanced by occasional supplementation with vitamin K, or by occasionally eating liver or broccoli.

Abram Hoffer's research was instrumental in getting niacin recognized as a heart protective drug, but nearly everyone who prescribes it does so to lower blood lipids. That was not Hoffer's understanding of its function. He thought it acted directly on blood vessels to protect their integrity. During his studies of its effects on heart disease, he saw that it also lowered cancer mortality, and so began treating cancer patients with it, with considerable success, but there was no medical cliché that could allow the profession to follow in that direction.

The arguments I have outlined for considering rosacea to be essentially a problem of metabolic energy, and the mechanisms that I mention for restoring mitochondrial functions, might seem more complex than Hoffer's orthomolecular views. However, this approach is actually much simpler conceptually than any of the ideologies of drug treatment. It simply points out that certain excitatory factors can interfere with energy production, and that there are opposing "inhibitory" factors that can restore energy efficiency. Sometimes, using just one or two of the factors can be curative.

Because mitochondrial respiration is very similar in every kind of tissue, a physiological view of rosacea could incline us toward considering the effects of these metabolic factors in other organs during stress and aging--what would the analogous condition of rosacea and rhinophyma be in the brain, heart, liver, or kidney?

References

Anisimov VN; Okulov VB. Probl Endokrinol (Mosk), 1981 Mar-Apr, 27:2, 48-52. [Blood estradiol level and G2-chalone content in the vaginal mucosa in rats of different ages] Batey DW, Eckhert CD. Invest Ophthalmol Vis Sci. 1991 Jun;32(7):1981-5.

Bellomio S. Boll Ocul. 1955 Mar;34(3):157-70. [Clinical contribution on riboflavin deficiency of the eye.] [Article in Italian]

Bertollo CM, Oliveira AC, Rocha LT, Costa KA, Nascimento EB Jr, Coelho MM. Eur J Pharmacol. 2006 Oct 10;547(1-3):184-91. Characterization of the antinociceptive and anti-inflammatory activities of riboflavin in different experimental models.

Blinova LI, Tsypin LM, Sheinberg AI. Vestn Oftalmol. 1961 Nov-Dec;74:48-53. [The content of riboflavin and ascorbic acid in the cornea in burns of the eye.] [Article in Russian]

Cardenas A, Moro MA, Hurtado O, Leza JC, Lorenzo P, Castrillo A, Bodelon OG, Bosca L, Lizasoain I. J Neurochem. 2000 May;74(5):2041-8. Implication of glutamate in the expression of inducible nitric oxide synthase after oxygen and glucose deprivation in rat forebrain slices.

Chan ES, Montesinos MC, Fernandez P, Desai A, Delano DL, Yee H, Reiss AB, Pillinger MH,

Chen JF, Schwarzschild MA, Friedman SL, Cronstein BN. Br J Pharmacol. 2006 Aug;148(8):1144-55. Adenosine A(2A) receptors play a role in the pathogenesis of hepatic cirrhosis.

Cutolo M, Capellino S, Montagna P, Villaggio B, Sulli A, Seriolo B, Straub RH. Clin Exp Rheumatol. 2003 Nov-Dec;21(6):687-90. New roles for estrogens in rheumatoid arthritis. Eikvar L, Kirkebøen KA. Tidsskr Nor Laegeforen. 1998 Mar 30;118(9):1390-5. [Receptormediated effects of adenosine and caffeine] [Article in Norwegian]

Engel A, Johnson ML, Haynes SG. Arch Dermatol. 1988 Jan;124(1):72-9. Health effects of sunlight exposure in the United States. Results from the first National Health and Nutrition Examination Survey, 1971-1974.

Funatsu H, Motegi T. Nippon Ganka Gakkai Zasshi. 1961 Dec 10;65:2439-44. [The effects of vitamin B2 group on the corneal metabolism. I.] [Article in Japanese]

Gehring W. J Cosmet Dermatol. 2004 Apr;3(2):88-93. Nicotinic acid/niacinamide and the skin.

Geng Y, Hansson GK, Holme E. Circ Res. 1992 Nov;71(5):1268-76. Interferon-gamma and tumor necrosis factor synergize to induce nitric oxide production and inhibit mitochondrial respiration in vascular smooth muscle cells.

Gordon OE. Q Bull Northwest Univ Med Sch. 1952;26(2):120-3. Riboflavin and the cornea.

Gougerot H, Grupper C, Plas G. Bull Soc Fr Dermatol Syphiligr. 1950 May-Jun;57(3):277-80. Cutaneous-mucosal ariboflavinosis; rosacea of cornea and medio-facial seborrheic dermatitis.

Gupta MA, Gupta AK, Chen SJ, Johnson AM. Br J Dermatol. 2005 Dec;153(6):1176-81. Comorbidity of rosacea and depression: an analysis of the National Ambulatory Medical Care Survey and National Hospital Ambulatory Care Survey--Outpatient Department data collected by the U.S. National Center for Health Statistics from 1995 to 2002.

Humphries KM, Szweda LI. Biochemistry. 1998 Nov 10;37(45):15835-41. Selective inactivation of alpha-ketoglutarate dehydrogenase and pyruvate dehydrogenase: reaction of lipoic acid with 4-hydroxy-2-nonenal.

Humphries KM, Yoo Y, Szweda LI. Biochemistry. 1998 Jan 13;37(2):552-7. Inhibition of NADH-linked mitochondrial respiration by 4-hydroxy-2-nonenal.

Irinoda K, Sato S. Tohoku J Exp Med. 1954 Dec 25;61(1):93-104. Contribution to the ocular manifestation of riboflavin deficiency.

Ishiwata T, Saito T, Hasegawa H, Yazawa T, Kotani Y, Otokawa M, Aihara Y. Brain Res. 2005 Jun 28;1048(1-2):32-40. Changes of body temperature and thermoregulatory responses of freely moving rats during GABAergic pharmacological stimulation to the preoptic area and anterior hypothalamus in several ambient temperatures.

Jarjour IT, Jarjour LK. Pediatr Neurol. 2005 Aug;33(2):94-7. Migraine and recurrent epistaxis in children.

Jefcoate CR, Liehr JG, Santen RJ, Sutter TR, Yager JD, Yue W, Santner SJ, Tekmal R, Demers L, Pauley R, Naftolin F, Mor G, Berstein L J Natl Cancer Inst Monogr 2000;(27):95-112. Tissue-specific synthesis and oxidative metabolism of estrogens.

Johnson ML, Grazul-Bilska AT, Redmer DA, Reynolds LP. Endocrine. 2006 Dec;30(3):333-42. Effects of estradiol-17beta on expression of mRNA for seven angiogenic factors and their receptors in the endometrium of ovariectomized (OVX) ewes.

Kendall SN. Clin Exp Dermatol. 2004 May;29(3):297-9. Remission of rosacea induced by reduction of gut transit time.

Koo SW, Hirakawa S, Fujii S, Kawasumi M, Nghiem P. Br J Dermatol. 2007 May;156(5):957-64. Protection from photodamage by topical application of caffeine after ultraviolet irradiation.

Lanari A, de Kremer GH. Medicina (B Aires) 1985;45(2):110-6. [Fibrosis and cirrhosis in the rabbit induced by diethylstilbestrol and its inhibition with progesterone]. [Article in Spanish]

Lovell MA, Xie C, Markesbery WR. Free Radic Biol Med. 2000 Oct 15;29(8):714-20. Acrolein, a product of lipid peroxidation, inhibits glucose and glutamate uptake in primary neuronal cultures.

Meno JR, Nguyen TS, Jensen EM, Alexander West G, Groysman L, Kung DK, Ngai AC, Britz GW, Winn HR. J Cereb Blood Flow Metab. 2005 Jun;25(6):775-84. Effect of caffeine on cerebral blood flow response to somatosensory stimulation.

Merighi S, Benini A, Mirandola P, Gessi S, Varani K, Simioni C, Leung E, Maclennan S, Baraldi PG, Borea PA. Mol Pharmacol. 2007 Aug;72(2):395-406. Caffeine inhibits adenosine-induced accumulation of hypoxia-inducible factor-1alpha, vascular endothelial growth factor, and interleukin-8 expression in hypoxic human colon cancer cells.

Moro MA, De Alba J, Cardenas A, De Cristobal J, Leza JC, Lizasoain I, Diaz-Guerra MJ, Bosca L, Lorenzo P. Neuropharmacology. 2000 Apr 27;39(7):1309-18. Mechanisms of the neuroprotective effect of aspirin after oxygen and glucose deprivation in rat forebrain slices.

Musey VC, Collins DC, Musey PI, Martino-Saltzman D, Preedy JR. Am J Obstet Gynecol 1987 Aug;157(2):312-317. Age-related changes in the female hormonal environment during reproductive life.

Nanji AA, Zakim D, Rahemtulla A, Daly T, Miao L, Zhao S, Khwaja S, Tahan SR, Dannenberg AJ. Hepatology. 1997 Dec;26(6):1538-45. Dietary saturated fatty acids down-regulate cyclooxygenase-2 and tumor necrosis factor alfa and reverse fibrosis in alcohol-induced liver disease in the rat.

Nishikawa M, Kimura S, Akaike N. J Physiol. 1994 Feb 15;475(1):83-93. Facilitatory effect of docosahexaenoic acid on N-methyl-D-aspartate response in pyramidal neurones of rat cerebral cortex.

Parkening TA; Lau IF; Saksena SK; Chang MC. J Gerontol, 1978 Mar, 33:2, 191-6. Circulating plasma levels of pregnenolone, progesterone, estrogen, luteinizing hormone, and follicle stimulating hormone in young and aged C57BL/6 mice during various stages of pregnancy.

Parola M, Bellomo G, Robino G, Barrera G, Dianzani MU. Antioxid Redox Signal. 1999 Fall;1(3):255-84. 4-Hydroxynonenal as a biological signal: molecular basis and pathophysiological implications.

Payne WG, Wang X, Walusimbi M, Ko F, Wright TE, Robson MC. Ann Plast Surg. 2002 Jun;48(6):641-5. Further evidence for the role of fibrosis in the pathobiology of rhinophyma.

Payne WG, Ko F, Anspaugh S, Wheeler CK, Wright TE, Robson MC. Ann Plast Surg. 2006 Mar;56(3):301-5. Down-regulating causes of fibrosis with tamoxifen: a possible cellular/molecular approach to treat rhinophyma.

Pellerin L, Wolfe LS. Neurochem Res. 1991 Sep;16(9):983-9. Release of arachidonic acid by NMDA-receptor activation in the rat hippocampus.

Picklo MJ, Amarnath V, McIntyre JO, Graham DG, Montine TJ. J Neurochem. 1999 Apr;72(4):1617-24. 4-Hydroxy-2(E)-nonenal inhibits CNS mitochondrial respiration at multiple sites.

Picklo MJ, Montine TJ. Biochim Biophys Acta. 2001 Feb 14;1535(2):145-52. Acrolein inhibits respiration in isolated brain mitochondria.

Prenen M, Ledoux-Corbusier M. Arch Belg Dermatol Syphiligr. 1971 Jul-Sep;27(3):253-8. [Hormonal contraception and dermatology]

Pu LL, Smith PD, Payne WG, Kuhn MA, Wang X, Ko F, Robson MC. Ann Plast Surg. 2000 Nov;45(5):515-9. Overexpression of transforming growth factor beta-2 and its receptor in rhinophyma: an alternative mechanism of pathobiology.

Randleman, MD, Assistant Professor, Department of Ophthalmology, Cornea, External Disease, and Refractive Surgery Section, Emory University School of Medicine

Rendl M, Mayer C, Weninger W, Tschachler E. Br J Dermatol. 2001 Jul;145(1):3-9. Topically applied lactic acid increases spontaneous secretion of vascular endothelial growth factor by human reconstructed epidermis.

Rivlin RS, Wolf G. Nature. 1969 Aug 2;223(5205):516-7. Diminished responsiveness to thyroid hormone in riboflavin-deficient rats.

Ryzhov S, McCaleb JL, Goldstein AE, Biaggioni I, Feoktistov I. J Pharmacol Exp Ther. 2007 Feb;320(2):565-72. Role of adenosine receptors in the regulation of angiogenic factors and neovascularization in hypoxia.

Santoro N, Brown JR, Adel T, Skurnick JH. J Clin Endocrinol Metab 1996 Apr;81(4):1495-501, Characterization of reproductive hormonal dynamics in the perimenopause.

Sibenge S, Gawkrodger DJ. J Am Acad Dermatol. 1992 Apr;26(4):590-3. Rosacea: a study of clinical patterns, blood flow, and the role of Demodex folliculorum.

Simkova M. Cesk Oftalmol. 1951;7(1):37-42. [Effect of vitamin B1 and B2 on diseases of the cornea.]

Simon N, Jolliet P, Morin C, Zini R, Urien S, Tillement JP. FEBS Lett. 1998 Sep 11;435(1):25-8. Glucocorticoids decrease cytochrome c oxidase activity of isolated rat kidney mitochondria.

Stern JJ. Am J Ophthalmol. 1950 Jul;33(7):1127-36. The ocular manifestations of riboflavin deficiency.

Stern HJ. Arch Ophthal. 1949 Oct;42(4):438-42. Conditioned corneal vascularity in riboflavin deficiency; report of a case.

Taketani T. Nippon Ganka Kiyo. 1962 Nov;13:489-94. [Variations of total vitamin B2 content in the cornea, iris and ciliary body and the blood of rabbits in stress. (A preliminary report)] [Article in Japanese]

Ullrich O, Henke W, Grune T, Siems WG. Free Radic Res. 1996 Jun;24(6):421-7. The effect of the lipid peroxidation product 4-hydroxynonenal and of its metabolite 4-hydroxynonenoic acid on respiration of rat kidney cortex mitochondria.

Wang YS, White TD. J Neurochem. 1999 Feb;72(2):652-60. The bacterial endotoxin lipopolysaccharide causes rapid inappropriate excitation in rat cortex.

Wiesinger H, Kaunitz H, Slanetz CA. Ophthalmologica. 1955 Jun;129(6):389-95. [Corneal changes in riboflavin-deficient rats.] [Article in German]

Wilhelmi G, Gdynia R. Arzneimittelforschung 1968 Dec;18(12): 1525-9. On the phlogogenic properties of lactic acid in animal experiments.

Wilkin JK. Ann Intern Med 1981 Oct;95(4):468-76. Flushing reactions: consequences and mechanisms.

Wilshire GB, Loughlin JS, Brown JR, Adel TE, Santoro N. J Clin Endocrinol Metab 1995 Feb;80(2):608-613. Diminished function of the somatotropic axis in older reproductive-aged women.

Yu AC, Chan PH, Fishman RA. J Neurochem 1986 Oct;47(4):1181-9. Effects of arachidonic acid on glutamate and gamma-aminobutyric acid uptake in primary cultures of rat cerebral cortical astrocytes and neurons.

Zaun H. Med Monatsschr Pharm. 1981 Jun;4(6):161-5. [Skin changes from taking hormonal contraceptives] [Article in German]

Psychological Stress and Rosacea

DAPHNE SU AND PROFESSOR PETER D. DRUMMOND, PH.D.

School of Psychology, Murdoch University, Perth, Western Australia, 6150, Australia
p.drummond@murdoch.edu.au

It has long been thought that rosacea is induced by emotional dysregulation. For instance, Klaber (1947) and Klaber & Wittkower (1939) asserted that feelings such as guilt, shame and social anxiety played a major role in the aetiology of rosacea. Others have suggested that frequent blushing may contribute to loss of contractile power in blood vessels, hence causing an increase in blood flow to the facial area (Miller, 1921; Klaber & Whittkower, 1939). However, many rosacea sufferers report being embarrassed by their condition and, as a result, blush easily. Whether this propensity to blush precedes the development of rosacea is unclear.

In addition to having to endure unpleasant symptoms, many rosacea sufferers report that prominent facial blemishes, together with stinging and burning sensations, can impact on their self-esteem and quality of life. Moreover, anxiety and depressive disorders are prevalent in patients with skin disorders, including rosacea (Harlow, Poyner, Finlay & Dykes, 2000; Gupta, 2005).

Current understanding of the link between psychological stress and rosacea is reviewed below. We begin with an overview of the relationship between stress and skin disorders, then examine physiological and emotional mechanisms of facial flushing and blushing. Finally, research on psychological well-being and skin conditions is addressed.

The Relationship between Stress and Skin Disorders

Various studies have reported an association between stress and certain skin disorders. Psoriasis, for instance, appears to be exacerbated by high stress levels. While the main function of the skin is to provide a flexible and protective shield against external stimuli, it also contains elements of the immune and nervous systems. Importantly, emotional state can influence cellular immune functions and neural discharge. Under stressful conditions, the skin reacts to activation of the hypothalamic-pituitary adrenal axis, subsequently affecting the regulation of stress hormones such as corticotropin-releasing hormone (CRH) and adrenocorticotropin (ACTH). Specifically, acute stress is associated with an increase in skin content of CRH (Theoharides et al., 2004). This activates mast cells, triggering inflammation.

Cutaneous mast cells are present in the vicinity of blood vessels and nerve terminals. When activated, mast cells release histamine, causing vasodilatation (Arck, Slominski, Theoharides, Peters, & Paus, 2005). Due to their close proximity to nerve terminals, mast cells may also be activated by antidromic discharge of C-fibres and secretion of substance P (a neuropeptide), which escalates the inflammation process further (Arck et al., 2005; Gee, Lynn & Cotsell, 1997). Hence, stress-induced cutaneous responses could create a vicious cycle of inflammation and heightened stress. Although the exact process by which stress impacts on rosacea is unclear, it is interesting to note that ondansetron, an oral medication used to treat rosacea, appears to reduce the incidence and intensity of flushing (Wollina, 1999). Ondansetron may block flushing by inhibiting release of substance P, possibly reducing the inflammatory process (Wollina, 1999).

Physiological Mechanisms of Facial Flushing and Blushing

Blushing is generally confined to the facial cutaneous region, namely the cheeks, forehead, chin, eyes, and neck, although it extends to the upper chest for some people. The vascular structure of this region is believed to differ from the other parts of the body, as capillary loops are much denser than normal and unusually close to the skin surface (Crozier, 2006; Wilkin, 1988). This concentration of shallow blood vessels in a small region allows greater blood flow to the cheek areas, resulting in the increased redness in the facial skin commonly observed during flushing or blushing episodes.

The sympathetic pathways that mediate thermoregulatory responses also control blood flow to the blush region (Drummond, 1997; Drummond, 1999a; Rothman, 1945; Rowell, 1977). For example, in an investigation of 23 patients, each with a lesion along the sympathetic pathway to the face, flushing and sweating were impaired on the denervated side of the forehead and cheek both during body heating and during embarrassment. The role of the sympathetic pathways in controlling facial flushing was further clarified by Drummond & Finch (1989), who found that thermoregulatory responses were reduced in the forehead and cheek during pharmacological blockade of the stellate ganglion. Blood flow was greater on the intact than blocked side during body heating, indicating that facial flushing was mediated by active sympathetic vasodilatation. In another report, a 32-year-old woman experienced a significant reduction of redness and burning sensations on her left cheek after the removal of two sympathetic ganglia, thus reiterating the role of sympathetic pathways in vasodilatation in the blush region. Evidence for sympathetic nervous system involvement in frequent blushing has also come from endoscopic transthoracic sympathectomy – a surgical procedure where a sympathetic nerve is cut or a sympathetic ganglion is removed to reduce sympathetic activity. In addition to sympathetic neural discharge, activation of beta-adrenergic receptors in the blood vessel wall by circulating catecholamines may contribute to flushing (Drummond, 1997).

A combination of vasoactive agents, neural activity and vascular structure can also influence blood flow to the facial region (Charkoudian, 2003). A reduction in the release of the sympathetic neurotransmitter noradrenaline induces vasodilatation of facial blood vessels. The release of noradrenaline and other vasoconstrictive neurotransmitters may be influenced by hormones circulating in the bloodstream. For instance, the flush observed in menopausal women is largely due to estrogen deficiency. The absence of this hormone seems to alter the release of various vasoconstrictors, thereby promoting active vasodilator function.

Other factors include the presence of vasodilators and consumption of certain food and beverages. Substances such as histamine, serotonin and vasoactive intestinal polypeptide can cause vasodilation by relaxing the muscle wall of facial blood vessels. Consumption of food, beverages and alcohol containing tyramine, monosodium glutamate, nitrites and sulfites may also influence vasodilatation. Furthermore, consumption of spicy food is known to increase body temperature and, in turn, invoke flushing reactions and local trigeminal-parasympathetic vasodilatation (Drummond, 1995).

Emotional Factors associated with Blushing and Flushing

Besides neural, immune and hormonal influences, strong emotions such as anger, guilt, shame, excitement, fear and embarrassment can trigger blushing (Darwin 1872/1998). This section examines the function of blushing, followed by a review of emotional influences on facial blood flow which focuses on the distress that individuals may face due to severe or prolonged blushing.

The Function of Blushing

Blushing, a fairly common physiological reaction, is thought to arise when people experience unwanted attention. Darwin (1872/1998) noted in his early writing that blushing is evident in individuals who experience strong emotions, and went further to question the function of blushing. Crozier (2006) reasoned that emotional blushing has social implications and its function is to correct social mistakes to assist in repairing relationships.

The notion that blushing is a mechanism to assist in mending relationships was explored by Semin & Manstead (1981). They investigated people's blushing reactions to an embarrassing incident, such as knocking over cans in a supermarket, and found that passers-by were more forgiving towards individuals who seemed embarrassed. Some individuals, however, experience great distress during frequent episodes of blushing and consider blushing to be an undesirable reaction in social situations. For these individuals, the distress may be great enough to lead them to develop a blushing phobia. Individuals with this fear often worry that others will notice their red face and criticise or give them negative comments.

Blushing Studies

Darwin (1872/1998) noted that blushing appears to be unique to humans. He suggested that blushing is a result of attention directed to the face and chest region, increasing blood flow to these areas. Studies on blushing have focused on understanding the possible physiological and emotional causes of the phenomenon.

Different instruments and physiological data have been used to investigate blushing. Some of the questionnaires developed included Leary and Meadows' (1991) questionnaire which required respondents to predict their own tendency to blush in different social scenarios, and Watson & Friend's (1969) questionnaire that measured respondents' anxiety level in social situations. Besides questionnaires, researchers have also measured physiological indicators of blushing. They include the use of laser Doppler flowmetry to measure skin blood flow (Drummond, 1997), a photoplethysmograph to measure blood pulse volume, thermistors to measure facial temperature, and other psychophysiological devices to measure emotional arousal.

The measurement of blushing poses numerous challenges; it is unlikely that accurate information can be obtained from a single source. For instance, blushing will be more easily detected in a person with fair complexion. But such observations are subjective and do not provide important information about the observer's own understanding of an observed blush reaction. On the other hand, self-perception measurements alone do not reflect physiological arousal. But taken together, these different measurements are able to provide a deeper understanding of blushing. Physiological measurements of blushing have shown fairly consistent patterns, demonstrating physiological arousal during blush-inducing circumstances (Mulkens et al., 1997; Mulkens et al., 1999). Several physiological indicators share common elements with emotions such as anxiety (Gerlach et al., 2001), anger and fear (Darwin, 1872/1998).

Blushing is a common phenomenon in humans. Not surprisingly, on Leary and Meadow's (1991) Blushing Propensity Scale (BPS), most participants thought that they blushed whenever they felt embarrassed. Participants perceived themselves to be blushing in a variety of scenarios, including being caught doing something inappropriate or improper, being the centre of attention and receiving positive attention such as praise. Participants also indicated that they rarely blushed while alone. This implied that one of the strongest elicitors of blushing was concern about what other people thought of them. Interestingly, the authors reported that high scorers on the BPS often scored highly on various aspects of social anxiety. These findings have since been replicated (Bögels, Alberts, & de Jong, 1996; Drummond, 1997; Mulkens, de Jong & Bögels, 1997; Neto, 1996).

It is not surprising that fear of blushing is often characterised by fear of negative evaluation. Individuals with this fear often report worrying that others will notice that they are blushing and criticise or give them negative comments. Watson & Friend (1969) found a positive relationship between social anxiety and fear of negative evaluation. Similarly, a study looking at fears and symptoms in social situations found statements such as "fear that others might notice the reactions" and "fears of looking nervous and insecure" were rated more frequently than other items in their questionnaire. In fact, blushing and trembling appear to be the most frequently experienced symptoms of anxiety in social situations.

Theories of blushing are centred on anxiety maintained by cognition and past learning experiences. For instance, Spector et al. (2003) reported that social phobics are hypervigilant to criticism as well as being conscious of their blushing being noticed by others. Similarly, Bögels & Lamers (2002) reported that social phobics are likely to overestimate negative social experiences and exaggerate potential negative consequences arising from them. In an experimental study, Mulkens et al. (1999) sought to understand the relationship between blushing propensity and estimation of blushing in fearful individuals and a control group. Interestingly, although physiological indicators (e.g., cheek temperature) did not reveal any differences between the two groups, individuals with a fear of blushing were more likely to report that they blushed intensely. This finding fitted the cognitive explanation of blushing phobia which posits that fear of blushing is maintained by ruminating thoughts on negative evaluation.

Past learning experiences may also play a part in maintaining a fear of blushing. Individuals with a fear of blushing often report negative blushing experiences such as being teased or bullied as children. The question remains, however, whether they were already anxious about blushing before those incidents or whether they had a tendency to pay more attention to negative events when they happened. Miller (2001) suggested that people become embarrassed because they vividly imagine what others might think of them. He also believed that childhood experiences such as being teased helped shape the responses to these emotions. Therefore, these people routinely overestimate the negative opinion of others towards themselves.

Recently, findings from physiological studies have highlighted the relationship between an individual's blushing propensity and past learning experiences. In particular, feedback to participants appears to influence self-reported blushing ratings. Drummond et al. (2003) attempted to induce embarrassment in 56 female undergraduates by asking them to sing in front of an experimenter, while measuring their facial blood flow. Participants were then informed by a female investigator about whether or not they had blushed while singing. Interestingly, increases in facial blood flow to the cheeks were found in participants with high blushing propensity scores who were told that they had "blushed". Disconfirming expectations of blushing (i.e., when participants were told that they were not blushing) seemed to inhibit facial blood flow even in high scorers on the BPS. The strongest effects of feedback, however, were on ratings of embarrassment – particularly following "blushing" feedback.

Physiological studies also point to the role of anxiety in individuals with a fear of blushing. Gerlach et al. (2001) investigated the physiological and psychological aspects of blushing and other somatic disorders. To induce embarrassment and blushing, participants were asked to sing a children's song while being videotaped. The participants were also informed that they would watch the videotape together with a small audience later on. Facial blood flow did not differ between social phobics with or without a primary concern about blushing. Interestingly, an increase in heart rate seemed to be the distinguishing factor between social phobics with and without the fear of blushing.

The role of anxiety has been further supported by Drummond (2001). Female participants were told to sing and read out loud. The tasks were divided into three categories where participants received accurate, false or no feedback via an auditory feedback signal. Despite being given negative feedback about blushing, high scorers on the BPS still blushed when they first sang whereas low scorers did not. Moreover, high scorers on the BPS rated themselves as highly embarrassed despite being told that they were not blushing. Taken together, it appears that participants focus on interoceptive sensations or cognitive cues in maintaining their fear.

Interestingly, many researchers have found no relationship between facial blood flow and blushing propensity scores, or even between physiological and self-reported measures of blushing during embarrassing encounters. For example, Mulkens et al. (1999) found women who scored highly on the BPS rated themselves as blushing more intensely than women with low scores. Physiologically, though, there was no difference in the cheek temperature between these groups. In an earlier experiment, Mulkens et al. (1997) found that irrespective of their scores on the BPS, cheek temperature increased while participants watched a videotape of themselves singing. However, high scorers were more concerned about their blushing than low scorers on the BPS. All in all, these findings suggest that an individual's self-perception of blushing intensity reflects his or her self-consciousness more closely than physiological reality.

Other studies have proposed that a slow recovery time could impact on fear of blushing. Drummond et al. (2003) found that facial blood flow increased progressively over the course of their study in participants with high BPS scores when they were told they were blushing after each consecutive task. In a more recent study, Drummond et al. (2007) found that blushing dissipated more slowly in participants with a fear of blushing. The authors suggested that an accumulative effect could have resulted in an overall increase in facial blood flow during the course of the study. Additionally, they suggested that a slow recovery from an episode of blushing might have resulted in physiological cues that maintained the fear of blushing. In sum, these findings suggest that a physiological predisposition, combined with a fear of negative evaluation, contributes to fear of blushing.

Emotional Influences on Flushing in Rosacea

Klaber and Wittkower (1939) reported that the majority of rosacea sufferers showed signs of social anxiety, indicating the involvement of a blushing phobia in rosacea sufferers. Rosacea sufferers often score highly on neuroticism scales (Whitlock, 1961; Marks, 1968). Whitlock (1961) in particular highlighted social anxiety as a concern for rosacea sufferers. Nonetheless, it is uncertain whether social anxiety develops before or after the onset of rosacea.

The majority of rosacea sufferers appear to have been childhood blushers. For instance, Klaber & Wittkower (1939) found that 33 of 50 rosacea sufferers had a history of childhood blushing compared with only 17 of 50 participants in the control group. In addition, Klaber and Wittkower (1939), Whitlock (1961) and Strokes, Beeman and Ingraham (1956) noted that rosacea sufferers often reported that social contact would elicit anxiety symptoms and increase the chance of a rosacea flushing episode. However, the physiological mechanisms that might be involved are unknown.

Psychological Well-being

Western culture places a heavy emphasis on facial appearance. It is perhaps not surprising then, that research has shown that having a disfiguring skin condition may have a profound impact on psychological well-being. While it is unclear whether rosacea is exacerbated by emotional factors, some early studies noted that some rosacea sufferers are likely to present with psychological symptoms.

Left untreated, co-morbid psychiatric disorders may impact adversely on quality of life (Gupta & Gupta, 2003). Furthermore, emotional stress is known to aggravate inflammatory skin disorders, including psoriasis, eczema and rosacea. Fortunately, appropriate psychological interventions appear to assist in the management of psychological distress and may help in the management of dermatological symptoms. With this in mind, the link between psychological well-being and skin disorders is reviewed in the following section. Intervention options are then discussed.

Psychological Well-being and Skin Disorders

Extensive research has been conducted on psychological well-being in patients with skin disorders (Bickers et al., 2006; Fleischer & Chen, 2005; Gupta, 2005; Gupta & Gupta, 2003; Hashiro & Okunura, 1997; Koo & Lebwohl, 2001; Madulika, Gupta & Gupta, 1996). Many have concluded that coping with a facial skin condition is difficult. In addition to physical discomfort, the development of a disfiguring skin disorder can have a negative impact on self-esteem, potentially leading to other psychiatric conditions. Psychiatric co-morbidity in dermatological disorders is well recognised. In many cases, the prevalence of psychiatric disorders, particularly mood and anxiety disorders (Bunker & Bridgett, 1997; Gupta, 2005; Gupta & Gupta, 1994; Gupta & Gupta, 2003), is reported to range between 25-30% of dermatological patients.

Depressive symptoms appear to be one of the most common psychological issues associated with dermatology disorders (Gupta, 2005; Picardi et al., 2004). According to the American Psychiatric Association (2000) and the National Centre for Classification in Health (2002), depression is associated with at least 2 weeks of depressed mood, and loss of interest in activities previously found enjoyable. Additionally, fatigue, loss of energy, a sense of hopelessness and recurrent thoughts of death may be experienced. In a number of skin disorders, a sense of hopelessness and lack of treatment response is associated with depression (Gupta, 2005; Gupta, Gupta & Johnson, 2005; Kimball, Jacobson, Weiss, Vreeland & Wu, 2005; Picardi et al., 2000). Furthermore, many dermatological patients encounter stigmatisation such as verbal rejection and stares due to disfigurement (Kent, 2005). Stigmatisation can affect the way dermatological patients view themselves mentally, severely impacting on their self esteem. In particular, skin disorders such as psoriasis (Gupta & Gupta, 1994; Kimball et al., 2005), atopic dermatitis and acne are frequently associated with depression.

Anxiety disorders, especially social anxiety and body dysmorphic disorder, are also frequently encountered in dermatological patients with disfiguring skin disorders (Gupta & Gupta, 2003; Picardi et al., 2004). Social phobia (American Psychiatric Association, 2000) is characterised by persistent fear and avoidance of social or performance situations where the individual may be exposed to possible scrutiny by others. Social anxiety may develop in conditions such as hyperhidrosis and rosacea, where sweating and blushing are prominent in embarrassing situations. Body dysmorphic disorder presents as a preoccupation with an imagined defect in appearance (American Psychiatric Association, 2000). Many individuals with body dysmorphic disorder experience distress over their "defect" which may lead to occupational and social difficulties (Gupta & Gupta, 2003). For many individuals with facial skin disfigurement, the fear of scrutiny, criticism and obsession with appearance is real. In an American study, Phillips et al. (2000) reported that approximately 12% of 268 dermatological patients met the criteria for body dysmorphic disorder. Given the disabling effects of social anxiety and body dysmorphic disorder, these conditions should be taken into consideration when treating skin conditions.

In addition to depression and anxiety disorders, quality of life is also known to be affected by dermatological disorders. Quality of life is defined as an individual's perception of life and potential to achieve his/her goals. Quality of life measurements enable dermatologists and other doctors to understand the impact of skin disorders on individual patients. Questions pertaining to unpleasant symptoms and feelings of self-consciousness are asked. Skin disorders such as eczema and psoriasis are associated with adverse scores on the Dermatology Quality of Life Questionnaire, indicating that skin conditions can impact significantly on quality of life.

Rosacea and Mental Health

Unfortunately, only a few studies have investigated the impact of rosacea on psychological well-being. While historically, emotional disorders were thought to have caused rosacea, case studies indicated that rosacea sufferers often described intensified social anxiety and depressive symptoms following their diagnosis (Whitlock, 1961). Furthermore, the older genre of research often compared psychological well-being of rosacea sufferers with patients with other dermatologic conditions, hence underestimating the severity of symptoms.

The few research papers that have been published recently on this topic indicate that rosacea sufferers are likely to be psychologically distressed. For example, a small scale questionnaire study conducted by nurses reported that the severity of rosacea symptoms was associated with dissatisfaction with self-image. Similarly, in a study by Balkrishnan et al. (2006), 73 women with severe skin conditions, including rosacea, reported a fear of negative evaluation. The authors conducted their survey study in Wake Forest University School of Medicine, North Carolina. Dermatologists from the university's clinic referred their patients for participation in the study. Participants were asked to fill out a survey consisting of demographics, medical history, dermatologic history, co-morbid conditions, quality of life and fear of negative evaluation. Unfortunately, only 4% of their participants were diagnosed with rosacea, hence reducing the specificity of results.

Gupta, Gupta & Johnson (2005) conducted a large study of 13.9 million participants who visited dermatological clinics across America. The authors collected their data from the National Ambulatory Medical Care Survey and the National Hospital Ambulatory Care Survey databases. Survey interviews were conducted by doctors or their staff. Information such as the nature of their visit and psychiatric diagnoses were tabulated. They reported that an estimated 4.81% of rosacea sufferers showed symptoms meeting the criteria of depression from the International Classification of Diseases version 9. Seventy percent of rosacea sufferers presenting with a co-morbid psychiatric diagnosis had depression. The authors argued that this figure was higher than the 29.9% prevalence of major depression for patients who attended psychiatric clinics in America. Apart from depression, there was no information regarding what the co-morbid psychiatric diagnoses were in this analysis. It is worth noting that subtypes and severity of rosacea were not included in the analysis; hence, it is unknown if particular subgroups of rosacea sufferers are more likely to be distressed by their condition.

Over the years, the National Rosacea Society of America has conducted informal online surveys. In 2007, 76% of 603 rosacea patients reported having low self-esteem, 69% said they felt embarrassed by the facial redness and disfigurement and 65% said they felt frustrated (http://www.rosacea.org/rr/2007/spring/article_3.php). While it is not known how severe their rosacea symptoms were, it cannot be denied that rosacea sufferers are indeed likely to show symptoms of psychological distress. In addition, rosacea appears to have an adverse effect on quality of life, with sufferers reporting that they avoid social interaction and experience feelings of embarrassment and self-consciousness (Abramova et al., 2004; de Belilovsky et al., 2007; Fleischer & Chen, 2005; Gupta & Chaudhry, 2003; Harlow et al., 2000). However, most quality of life surveys are limited by the small number of rosacea sufferers participating.

Psychological aspects of rosacea were reviewed by Garnis-Jones (1998) and Nase (2001). These articles highlight the importance of understanding and recognising psychological symptoms such as self-consciousness, anxiety and depression in rosacea. They further stress the importance of identifying the amount of distress the individual may be experiencing due to rosacea. A case study by Cohen et al. (1991) demonstrated the importance of early intervention and holistic management of the condition. A 36-year-old woman diagnosed with rosacea became preoccupied with her appearance. Unable to cope with her anxiety and depressive symptoms, she resigned from her job and attempted suicide. While the case study is extreme, Cohen et al. (1991) emphasised the importance of early detection of psychological distress by dermatologists and early referral for psychological intervention.

Psychological Intervention

Many researchers highlight the importance of managing rosacea with appropriate medication and psychological intervention (Bikowaski, 2000; Bikowaski & Goldman,

2004; Gupta & Chaudhry, 2005; Swinyer, 1994). To the best of our knowledge, no specific psychological intervention has been developed for rosacea sufferers. Fortunately, however, psychological interventions tailored to other skin disorders can assist in reducing psychological distress. In some cases, a combination of psychotropic medication and psychological intervention can relieve certain symptoms (Gupta & Gupta, 1996). Cognitive behavioural therapy, psychotherapy, behavioural therapy and group therapy were reported to assist dermatological patients cope with their condition. Providing information regarding their skin condition, counselling, relaxation therapy, assertiveness and social skills training are some examples of strategies that psychologists can use. Regardless of the medium of intervention, the goal is to assist dermatologic sufferers to identify useful coping strategies, examine difficulties and issues that they may be experiencing due to their condition, facilitate social interaction skills and provide emotional and social support.

The results of psychological intervention for dermatological conditions appear to be positive. A 12-week psychotherapy individual program consisting of relaxation training, imagery training and cognitive-behavioural stress management techniques for psoriasis sufferers led to significant reductions in stress levels (Zachariae et al., 1996). Moreover, the experimental group experienced a reduction in psoriasis symptoms, indicating better coping. Interestingly, laser Doppler flowmetry measurements of blood flow showed that relaxation and imagery training decreased blood flow during the session itself. This indicates that it is possible to affect blood flow in inflamed skin (Locke et al., 1994). The treatment of atopic dermatitis using cognitive behavioural therapy (Ehlers et al., 1995), psoriasis using mindfulness techniques (Kabat-Zinn et al., 1998), and social skills training in a group setting (Robinson et al., 1996) all achieved positive results.

Summary

As the experience of having a skin condition can be distressing, it is not surprising that psychological disorders such as anxiety and depression are prevalent in dermatological settings. While research in the area of rosacea is limited, the few papers published appear to indicate that rosacea sufferers, particularly individuals with severe symptoms, may experience psychological distress. Furthermore, while psychological intervention appears to be helpful for dermatological patients in general to better cope with their condition, more studies are needed to understand and evaluate the role of psychological intervention specifically for rosacea.

References

Abramova, L., Yeung, J., Chren, M. M., & Chen, S. (2004). Rosacea quality of life index (ROSAQOL). Journal of the American Academy of Dermatology, 50(3). P12.

American Psychiatric Association. (2000). Diagnostic and statistical manual of mental disorders (4th ed.). Washington, DC: American Psychiatric Association.

Arck, P. C., Slominski, A., Theoharides, T. C., Peters, E. M. J., Paus, R. (2006). Neuroimmunology of stress: Skin takes center stage. Journal of Investigative Dermatology, 126(8), 1697-1704.

Balkrishnan, R., McMichael, A. J., Hu, J. Y., Camacho, F. T., Shew, K. R., Bouloc, A., et al. (2006). Correlates of health-related quality of life in women with severe facial blemishes. The International Society of Dermatology, 45, 111-115.

Bickers, D. R., Lim, H. W., Margolis, D., Weinstock, M. A., Goodman, C., Faulkner, E., et al. (2006). The burden of skin diseases: 2004. Journal of the American Academy of Dermatology, 55, 490-500.

Bikowaski, J. B., & Goldman, M. P. (2004). Rosacea: Where are we now? Journal of Drugs in Dermatology, 3(3), 251-261.

Bögels, S. M., Alberts, M., & de Jong, P. J. (1996). Self consciousness, self focused attention, blushing propensity and fear of blushing. Personality and Individual Differences, 21, 573-581.

Bögels, S. M., & Lamers, C. T. J. (2002). The causal role of self-awareness in blushing-anxious, socially-anxious and social phobics individuals. Behaviour Research and Therapy, 40, 1367-1384.

Brazzini, B., Ghersetich, I., Hercogova, J., & Lotti, T. (2003). The neuro-immuno-cutaneous endocrine network: Relationship between mind and skin. Dermatologic Therapy, 16, 123-131.

Bunker, C., & Bridgett, C. K. (1997). Depression and the skin. In M. M. Robertson & C. L. E. Katona (Eds.), Depression and physical illness. West Sussex: John Wiley and Sons.

Burkhart, K. L., Shelestak, D., & Lappin, J. (2005). Perceptions of self in persons with rosacea. Dermatology Nursing, 17(4), 249-314. Callejas, M. A., Rubio, M., Iglesias, N., J., V., Canalís, E., Catalán, M., et al. (2004). Video-assisted thoracoscopic sympathectomy for the treatment of facial blushing: Ultrasonic scalpel versus diathermy. Archives of Bronconeumology, 40(1), 17-19.

Carroll, C. L., Balkrishnan, R., Feldman, S. R., Fleischer, A., & Manuel, J. C. (2005). The burden of atopic dermatitis: Impact on the patient, family, and society. Pediatric Dermatology, 22(3), 192-199.

Charkoudian, N. (2003). Skin blood flow in adult human thermoregulation: How it works, when it does not, and why. Mayo Clinic Proceedings, 78(5), 603-612.

Chiu, A., Chon, S. Y., & Kimball, A. B. (2003). The response of stress disease to stress. Archives of Dermatology, 139, 897-900.

Clark, D. M., Ehlers, A., Hackmann, A., McManus, F., & Fennel, M. (2006). Cognitive therapy versus exposure and applied relaxation in social phobia: A randomised controlled trial. Journal of Consulting and Clinical Psychology, 74(3), 568-578.

Cohen, C., Krahn, L., Wise, T. N., Epstein, S., & Ross, R. (1991). Delusions of disfigurement in a woman with acne rosacea. General Hospital Psychiatry, 13, 273-277.

Crozier, W. R. (2006). Blushing and the social emotions. New York: Palgrave Macmillan.

Darwin, C. (1872/1998). The expression of the emotions in man and animals (3rd ed.). New York: Oxford Press.

de Belilovsky, C., Fournier, A., & Pernet, A. M. (2007). Equale study: Impact of rosacea on quality of life of affected patients. Journal of the American Academy of Dermatology, 56(2), AB16.

Drummond, P. D., Back, K., Harrison, J., Helgadottir, F., Lange, B., Lee, C., et al. (2007). Blushing during social interactions in people with a fear of blushing. Behaviour Research and Therapy, 45, 1601-1608.

Drummond, P. D. (1995). Mechanisms of physiological gustatory sweating and flushing in the face. Journal of the Autonomic Nervous System, 52, 117-124.

Drummond, P. D. (1997a). The effect of adrenergic blockage and facial flushing. Psychophysiology, 34(2), 163-168.

Drummond, P. D. (1997b). Correlates of facial flushing and pallor in anger-provoking situations. Personality and Individual Differences, 23(4), 575-582.

Drummond, P. D. (1999a). Autonomic disorders affecting cutaneous blood flow. In C. J. Mathias & R. Bannister (Eds.), Autonomic failure. A textbook of clinical disorders of the autonomic nervous system (4th ed.). London: Oxford University Press.

Drummond, P. D. (1999b). Facial flushing during provocation in women. Psychophysiology, 36, 325-332.

Drummond, P. D. (2001). The effect of true and false feedback on blushing in women. Personality and Individual Differences, 30, 1329-1343.

Drummond, P. D., Camacho, L., Formentin, N., Heffernan, T. D., Williams, F., & Zekas, T. E. (2003). The impact of verbal feedback about blushing on social discomfort and facial blood flow during embarrassing tasks. Behavior Research and Therapy, 41, 413-425.

Drummond, P. D., & Finch, P. M. (1989). Reflex control of facial flushing during body heating in man. Brain, 112, 1351-1358.

Drummond, P. D., & Lance, J. W. (1987). Facial flushing and sweating mediated by the sympathetic nervous system. Brain, 110, 793-803.

Drummond, P. D., & Lim, H. K. (2000). The significance of blushing for fair- and dark-skinned people. Personality and Individual Differences, 29, 1123-1132.

Drummond, P. D., & Quah, S. H. (2001). The effect of expressing anger on cardiovascular reactivity and facial blood flow in Chinese and Caucasians. . Psychophysiology, 38, 190-196.

Ehlers, A., Stangier, U., Gieler, U., Grey, N., Waddington, L., & Wild, J. (1995). Treatment of atopic dermatitis: A comparison of psychological and dermatological approaches to relapse prevention. Journal of Consulting and Clinical Psychology, 63(4), 624-635.

Fahlén, T. (1996/1997). Core symptom pattern of social phobia. Depression and Anxiety, 4, 223-232.

Fleischer, A., & Chen, S. (2005). The face and mind evaluation study: An examination of the efficacy of rosacea treatment using physician ratings and patient self-reported quality of life. Journal of Drugs in Dermatology, 4(5), 585-590.

Finlay, A. Y. (1997). Quality of life measurement in dermatology: a practical guide. British Journal of Dermatology, 136(3), 305-314.

Garnis-Jones, S. (1998). Psychological aspects of rosacea. Journal of Cutaneous Medicine and Surgery, 2, 4-16.

Gerlach, A. L., Wihelm, F. H., Gruber, K., & Roth, W. T. (2001). Blushing and physiological arousability in social phobia. Journal of Abnormal Psychology, 110(2), 247-258.

Gupta, A. K., & Chaudhry, M. M. (2003). Critical review of the manner in which the efficacy of therapies for rosacea are evaluated. International Journal of Dermatology, 42, 909-916.

Gupta, A. K., & Chaudhry, M. M. (2005). Rosacea and its management: An overview. European Academy of Dermatology and Venereology, 19, 273-285.

Gupta, A. M. (2005). Psychiatric comorbidity in dermatologic disorders. In C. Walker & L. Papadopoulos (Eds.), Psychodermatology. The psychological impact of skin disorders (pp. 29-39). Cambridge: Cambridge.

Gupta, A. M., & Gupta, A. K. (1996). Psychodermatology: An update. Journal of the American Academy of Dermatology, 34(6), 1030-1046.

Gupta, M. A., & Gupta, A. (1994). Depression modulates pruritus perception: A study of pruritus in psoriasis, atopic dermatitis, and chronic idiopathic urticaria. Psychosomatic Medicine, 56, 36-40.

Gupta, M. A., & Gupta, A. K. (2003). Psychiatric and psychological co-morbidity in patients with dermatologic disorders. American Journal of Clinical Dermatology, 4(12), 833-842.

Gupta, M. A., Gupta, A. K., & Johnson, A. M. (2005). Comorbidity of rosacea and depression: An analysis of the National Ambulartory Medical Care Survey and National Hospital Ambulatory Care Survey-Outpatient department data collected by the U.S. National center of health statistics from 1995-2002. Epidemiology and Health Services Research, 153, 1176-1181.

Harlow, D., Poyner, T., Finlay, A. Y., & Dykes, P. J. (2000). Impaired quality of life of adults in skin disease in primary care. British Journal of Dermatology, 143, 979-982. Hashiro, M., & Okumura, M. (1997). Anxiety, depression and psychosomatic symptoms in patients with atopic dermatitis: Comparison with normal controls and among groups of different degrees of severity. Journal of Dermatological Science, 14, 63-67.

Izikson, L., English, J. C., & Zirwas, M. J. (2006). The flushing patient: Differential diagnosis, workup, and treatment. Journal of the American Academy of Dermatology, 55, 193-208.

Kabat-Zinn, J., Wheeler, E., Light, T., Skillings, A., Scharf, M., Cropley, T. G., et al. (1998). Influence of a mindfulness meditation-based stress reduction intervention on rates of skin clearing in patients with moderate to severe psoriasis undergoing phototherapy (UVB) and photochemotherapy (PUVA). Psychosomatic Medicine, 60, 625-632.

Kent, G. (2005). Stigmatisation and skin conditions. In C. Walker & L. Papadopoulos (Eds.), Psychodermatology: The psychological impact of skin disorders. New York: Cambridge University Press.

Kim, J. S., Kim, Y. J., Jim, T. Y., Song, J. Y., Cho, Y. H., Park, Y. C., et al. (2005). Association of ALDH2 polymorphism with sensitivity to acetaldehyde-induced micronuclei and facial flushing after alcohol intake. Toxicology, 210 (2-3), 169-174.

Kimball, A. B., Jacobson, C., Weiss, S., Vreeland, M. G., & Wu, Y. (2005). The psychosocial burden of psoriasis. American Journal of Clinical Dermatology, 6(6), 383-392.

Klaber, R. (1947). Psychological factors in the aetiology of certain skin diseases. The British Journal of Dermatology and Syphilis, 59, 1-6.

Klaber, R., & Wittkower, E. (1939). The pathogenesis of rosacea. The British Journal of Dermatology and Syphilis, LI, 501-519.

Kleve, L., Rumsey, N., Wyn-Williams, M., & White, P. (2002). The effectiveness of cognitive-behavioral interventions provided at Outlook: A disfigurement support unit. Journal of Evaluation in Clinical Practice, 8(4), 387-395.

Koo, J., & Lebwohl, A. (2001). Psychodermatology: The mind and skin connection. American Family Physician, 64(11), 1873-1878.

Leary, M. R., & Meadows, S. (1991). Predictors, elicitors, and concomitants of social blushing. Journal of Personality and Social Psychology, 60(2), 254-262.

Locke, S., Ransil, B., Zachariae, R., Molay, F., Tollins, K., Covino, N., et al. (1994). Effect of hypnotic suggestion on the delayed-type hypersensitivity response. The Journal of the American Medical Association, 372(1), 47-52.

Marks, R. (1968). Concepts in the pathogenesis of rosacea. British Journal of Dermatology, 80, 170-177.

Mazzotti, E., Picardi, A. Sampogna, F., Pasquini, P., & Abeni, D. (2003). Sensitivity of the dermatology quality of life index to clinical change in patients with psoriasis. British Journal of Dermatology, 149, 318-322.

Millard, L. (2000). Dermatological practice and psychiatry. British Journal of Dermatology, 143(5), 920-921.

Miller, F. P. (1921). Etiology of acne rosacea through a viscero-neurologic mechanism. American Journal of Medical Sciences, 161, 120-124.

Miller, R. S. (2001). Shyness and embarrassment compared: Siblings in the service of social evaluation, in W.R. Crozier and L.E. Alden (eds), International Handbook of Social Anxiety, Chichester, Sussex: Wiley, pp.281-300.

Mulkens, S., & Bögels, S. M. (1999). Learning history in fear of blushing. Behaviour Research and Therapy, 37, 1159-1167.

Mulkens, S., de Jong, P. J., & Bögels, S. M. (1997). High blushing propensity: Fearful preoccupation or facial coloration? Personality and Individual Differences, 22, 817-824.

Mulkens, S., de Jong, P. J., Dobbelaar, A., & Bögels, S. M. (1999). Fear of blushing: Fearful preoccupation irrespective of facial coloration. Behavior Research and Therapy, 37, 1119-1128.

Nase, G. (2001). Effect of depression and anxiety on rosacea. In G. Nase (Ed.), Beating rosacea: Vascular, ocular and acne forms. Indiana: Nase Publications.

National Centre for Classification in Health. (2002). International Statistical Classification of Diseases and Related Health Problems (10th ed.). Sydney: The University of Sydney.

National Rosacea Society. (2007). Survey shows Rosacea emotional toll, positive effects of medical therapy. Retrieved 6th August of 2008 from www.rosacea.org/rr/2007/spring/article_3.php.

Neto, F. (1996). Correlates of social blushing. Personality and Individual Differences, 20(3), 365-373.

O'Sullivan, R., Graema, L., & Lerner, E. (1998). The neuro-innuno-cutaneous-endocrine network: Relationship of mind and skin. Archives of Dermatology, 134(11), 1431-1435.

Papadopoulos, L. (2005). Psychological therapies for dermatological problems. In C. Walker & L. Papadopoulos (Eds.), Psychodermatology. The psychological impact of skin disorders. Cambridge: Cambridge University Press.

Papadopoulos, L., Walker, C., Aitken, D., & Bor, R. (2000). The relationship between body location and psychological morbidity in individuals with acne vulgaris. Psychology, Health & Medicine, 5(4), 431-438.

Phillips, K. A., Dufresne, R. G., Wilkel, C. S., & Wittoria, C. C. (2000). Rate of body dysmorphic disorder in dermatology patients. Journal of the American Academy of Dermatology, 42, 436-441.

Picardi, A., & Abeni, D. (2001). Stressful life events and skin diseases: Disentangling evidence from myth. Psychotherapy and Psychosomatics, 70(3), 118-136.

Picardi, A., Abeni, D., Melchi, C. F., Puddu, P., & Pasquini, P. (2000). Psychiatric morbidity in dermatological outpatients: An issue to be recognized. British Journal of Dermatology, 143, 983-991.

Picardi, A., Ameria, A., Baliva, G., Barbieri, C., Teofoli, P., Bolli, S., et al. (2004). Recognition of depressive and anxiety disorders in dermatological outpatients. Acta Dermato-Venereologica, 84, 213-217.

Robinson, E., Rumsey, N., & Partridge, J. (1996). An evaluation of the impact of social interaction skills training for facially disfigured people. British Journal of Plastic Surgery, 49, 281-286.

Rowell, L. B. (1977). Reflex control of the cutaneous vasculature. Journal of Investigative Dermatology, 69, 154-166.

Rothman, S. (1945). The role of autonomic nervous system in cutaneous disorders. Psychosomatic Medicine, 7(9), 90-96.

Saxen, M. A., & Campbell, R. L. (1995). An unusual case of sympathetically maintained facial pain complicated by telangiectasia. Oral Surgery, Oral Medicine, Oral Pathology, Oral Radiology, and Endodontology, 79(4), 455-458.

Semin, G. R., & Manstead, A. S. R. (1981). The beholder beheld: A study of social emotionality. European Journal of Social Psychology, 12, 367-377.

Shenefelt, P. D. (2006). Nondrug psychotherapeutic options for skin disorders. In M. E. Abelian (Ed.), Trends in psychotherapy research (pp. 33-51). New York: Nova Science Publishers

Spector, I. P., Pecknold, J. C., & Libman, E. (2003). Selective attentional bias related to the noticeability aspect of anxiety symptoms in generalised social phobia. Anxiety Disorders, 17, 517-531.

Stein, D. J., & Bouwer, C. (1997). Blushing and social phobia: A neuroethological speculation. Medical Hypotheses, 49, 101-108.

Stenberg, B., Eriksson, N., Hansson, K., Höög, J., Sandström, M., Sundell, J., et al. (1995). Facial skin symptoms in visual display terminal (VDT) workers. A case-referent study of personal, psychosocial, building-and VDT related risk indicators. International Journal of Epidemiology, 24(4), 796-803.

Strokes, J. H., Beerman, H., & Ingraham, N. R. (1956). A re-evaluation of the rosacea complex. American Journal of Medical Science, 232, 458-473.

Swinyer, T. (1994). Recognizing and managing rosacea. The American Journal of Nursing, 97(12), 16AAA-16DDD.

Theoharis, C., Donelan, J. M., Papadopoulou, N., Cao, J. Kempuraj, D., & Conti, P. (2004). Mast cells as targets of corticotropin-releasing factor and related peptides. Trends in Pharmacological Sciences, 25(11), 563-568.

Telaranta, T. (1998). Treatment of social phobia by endoscopic thoracic sympatheticotomy. European Journal of Surgery, 164, 27-32.

Watson, D., & Friend, R. (1969). Measurement of social-evaluative anxiety. Journal of Consulting and Clinical Psychology, 33(4), 448-457.

Webster, G. F. (2001). Acne vulgaris and rosacea: Evaluation and management. Office Dermatology, 4(1), 15-22.

Whitlock, F. A. (1961). Psychosomatic aspects of rosacea. British Journal of Dermatology, 73, 137-148.

Wilkin, J. K. (1988). Why is flushing limited to a mostly facial cutaneous distribution? Journal of American Academy of Dermatology, 19, 309-313.

Wilkin, J., Dahl, M., Detmar, M., Drake, L., Feinstein, A., Odom, R., et al. (2002). Standard classification of rosacea: Report of the National Rosacea Society Expert Committee on the classification and staging of rosacea. Journal of the American Academy of Dermatology, 46, 584-587.

Wilkin, J., Dahl, M., Detmar, M., Drake, L., Liang, M., Odom, R., et al. (2004). Standard grading system for rosacea: Report of the National Rosacea Society Expert Committee on the classification and staging of rosacea. Journal of the American Academy of Dermatology, 50, 907-912.

Wollina, U. (1999). The response to erthematous rosacea to ondanseton. British Journal of Dermatology, 140, 561-562.

Zachariae, R., Oster, H., Bjerring, P., & Kragballe, K. (1996). Effects of psychologic intervention of psoriasis. A preliminary report. Journal of the American Academy of Dermatology, 34, 1008-1015.

Zachariae, R., Zachariae, C., Ibsen, H., Mortensen, H. T., & Wulf, H. C. (2004). Psychological symptoms and quality of life of dermatology outpatients and hospitalized dermatology patients. Acta Dermato-Venereologica, 84, 205-212.

The Role of Demodex Mites in the Pathogenesis of Rosacea and Blepharitis and Their Control

KOSTA Y. MUMCUOGLU, PH. D.[1] AND OLEG E. AKILOV, M. D., PH.D.[2]

[1]Department of Microbiology and Molecular Genetics, The Kuvin Center for the Study of Infectious and Tropical Diseases, The Institute for Medical Research Israel-Canada, The Hebrew University - Hadassah Medical School, Jerusalem, Israel
kostam@cc.huji.ac.il
[2]Department of Dermatology, University of Pittsburgh, Pittsburgh, Pennsylvania, USA

The follicle mites *Demodex folliculorum* and *Demodex brevis* could play a role in several skin and ocular diseases; however, in lower numbers these mites could also be found in healthy individuals. Demodicosis is a chronic skin disease, which affects mainly the face and it is caused by the presence of large number of follicle mites. Rosacea complicated by Demodex mite infestation and Demodex blepharitis present therapeutic difficulties in everyday practice. Acaricidal formulations containing lindane, crotamiton, permethrin, sulfur, mercury and ivermectin have been shown to be effective in diminishing the number of mites and alleviating the symptoms of demodicosis.

Introduction

Demodicosis is a chronic skin disease, which affects mainly the face and it is caused by the follicle mites of the genus *Demodex*. The diagnosis of demodicosis is complicated by the fact that these mites are also found on the skin of healthy individuals. The rate of healthy carriers varies between 11.9% and 72.0% [1-3]. It has been suggested, however, that demodicosis develops only in predisposed people [4].

The aim of this review article was to summarize our knowledge in the etiopathological role of Demodex mites in the development of some forms of rosacea and blepharitis, and to discuss the treatment modalities in order to control the mites and treat symptoms of demodicosis.

Demodex and Rosacea

Kaufmann-Wolf [5] was the first to report in 1925 that *Demodex folliculorum* could be responsible for skin alterations such as rosacea. In 1930, Ayres [6] described a skin disease "pityriasis folliculorum" in women who used cosmetic preparations rather than soap and water for their daily facial skin care. Antiparasitic treatment and use of soap and water resulted in prompt cure. Ayres & Anderson [7] reported on 17 patients with a rosacea-like dermatosis, in whom *D. folliculorum* was found in milky vesicles and pustules or in follicular scales. Again, an antiparasitic treatment led to an improvement of the clinical manifestations with a parallel diminution in the number of mites.

Ayres & Ayres [8] reported 203 patients with "pityriasis folliculorum" and "acne rosacea of Demodex-type". The latter was described as a rosacea-like dermatosis of external origin, which is to be distinguished from rosacea by presence of small pustules, superficial granulomas, and oily skin. Demodex mites were recovered in great numbers from the superficial vesicles and pustules. Applications of "Danish ointment" led to disappearance of the mites and marked improvement or complete cure of the skin diseases. Russell [9] and Spickett [10] stressed the quantitative aspects and related the heaviness of infestation to the frequency of infested follicles or to the number of mites within such follicles.

Recently, different forms of atypical demodicosis such as unilateral demodicosis [11], demodicosis of the sebaceous glands of the oral mucosa [12], Demodex granuloma [13, 14], spinulosis of the face [15] and tubero-pustular demodicosis has been described [16]. New forms of this disease have been reported in HIV-infected individuals [17-20]. Akbulatova [21] observed six forms of demodicosis, i.e., oligosymptomatic, erythematic squamous, papulous, papulo-vesiculous, papulo-pustulous and mixed forms. Akilov et al [22] suggested that demodicosis could be divided into primary and secondary types, based on the development of the disease on previously healthy skin (primary process) or as a complication of pre-existing dermatoses such as perioral dermatitis and rosacea (secondary type). The usual etiological agent of primary demodicosis is *D. folliculorum*, which causes an erythemato-squamous eruption in the T-zone of the face. The efflorescence is always accompanied by a pruritus, which first could be noted with appearance of the first lesions. The inflammatory erythema, which starts after the vesico-papules have emerged, disappears after treatment. The secondary demodicosis is mainly caused by *D. brevis* and characterized by a papulo-pustulous eruption located symmetrically and predominately in the molar regions of the face. The efflorescence appears on an altered skin due to a dermatosis of different origin and involves larger areas of the face than primary demodicosis. The pruritus is not a constant feature and usually starts after the exacerbation of the lesion. The erythema exists before the papulo-pustular eruption, is due to abnormal vascular reactivity and continues after the treatment. Thus, it should be emphasized that demodicosis and rosacea are separate entities with sometimes similar clinical pictures. Demodex mite infestation may complicate an existing rosacea but this is almost always a secondary process (except in the case of Demodex granuloma / granulomatous rosacea, which are beyond the scope of this review).

Demodex blepharitis

Demodex blepharitis (also known as demodectic blepharitis, blepharitis palpebrarum and ocular demodicosis) has been known for a long time in the ophthalmologic literature and is well documented. Raehlmann first described this disease in 1899 [23]. Morgan & Coston [24] reported the case of 20 patients with isolated Demodex blepharitis. Burning and itching of the eyelids, redness, scaling, pigmentation about the roots of the cilia, cellular mantles about the basis of the cilia and conjunctival injection were the presenting features. Out of 18 patients with rosacea, 12 had Demodex mites in their eyelash follicles, while in 54 patients with seborrhea and seborrhoic dermatitis and in 30 patients with acne no mites were found in the ciliary follicles. Ayres & Mihan [25] also mentioned a Demodex blepharitis in the course of rosacea with high numbers of mite, which cleared under "Danish ointment". Post & Juhlin [26] described Demodex blepharitis as an inflammation of the lid margins with matted, irregularly growing, scanty and loose eye-lashes and an accumulation of debris at their base. Turk et al. [27] demonstrated *D. folliculorum* in 11 out of 37 (29.7%) patients with blepharitis, in 1 out of 11 (9.1%) patients with blepharo-conjunctivitis and in 2 out of 48 (4.2%) persons in the healthy control group.

Today, it is believed that the pathological changes in the course of demodicosis of the eyelids are consequences of: (1) blockage of follicles and leading out tubules of sebaceous glands by the mites and by reactive hyperkeratinization and epithelial hyperplasia; (2) a mechanical vector role of bacteria; (3) host's inflammatory reaction to the presence of parasite's chitin as a foreign body; (4) stimulation of the host's humoral responses and cell-mediated immunological reactions under the influence of mites and their waste products; (5) super-infection by Demodex, which often occurs in the course of chronic blepharitis; (6) age related changes; and (7) immunocompromised conditions. Treatment of demodicosis of the eyelids as a general rule takes a few months [28].

Demodex mites

The follicle mites, *D. folliculorum* and *D. brevis* are permanent ectoparasites of the skin, man being their exclusive host. Both species are found worldwide and have been recovered in all investigated racial groups of man [29].They are spindle-shaped; their body is practically hairless and colorless. They are 0.3-0.4 mm long and have 4 short pairs of legs, which are located on the anterior third of their body, while the posterior portion of the body shows a secondary striation. *D. folliculorum* is practically always found in the hair follicles of the nasolabial folds, the nose and the eyelids, while *D. brevis* is mainly living in the sebaceous glands. Both feed on cells of the follicular and sebaceous gland epithelium by perforating the cell wall with their piercing mouthparts and sucking the cell contents [30]. The greatest concentration of mites was found in sites where sebaceous glands are numerous and sebum production is pronounced. The transmission occurs by close contact between two individuals.

Detection of mites on the skin

For the detection of the mites on and in the skin different methods have been applied:
1. Isolating the mites with the help of adhesive tape strips, which are applied on and then removed from the skin.
2. Piercing the pustules with the help of a sterile needle.
3. Removing the content of the follicles with the help of a scalpel by squeezing the skin or with a comedone extractor.
4. Using the cyanoacrylate adhesive (also called skin surface biopsy), which penetrates the follicles and after solidification removes the follicle content.
5. Taking skin biopsies.

Treatment of Demodex mite infestation

The treatment of a patient with Demodex mite infestation depends on underlying skin process. For patients with history of rosacea and recent findings of Demodex mites, the first line therapy should be anti-rosacea medication. Surprisingly, Demodex mites can disappear after sufficient measures directed towards improvement of the pre-existing skin condition. In case of persistent Demodex mite infestation, acaricidal medications are needed, but in any case not as a first line treatment due to prominent local irritating effects, which can lead to eczematisation of the facial skin.

Different acaricidal medications are available. All of them are effective against Demodex; however, the spectrum of side effects influences their choice. Rufli et al. [31] treated 36 patients with rosacea with 0.25% hexachlorocyclohexane (lindane), 9 with 10% crotamiton emulsion and 6 with Unguentum hydrargyrum praecipitatum album (2%), all of which have acaricidal and insecticidal properties. Patients were treated once a day and the therapy lasted for 7 weeks, until all patients were free of symptoms. In the majority of patients who were treated with lindane, a local flare-up reaction accompanied by a burning sensation has been observed from the first day of the treatment, which lasted for 15-30 min and was observed during the first two weeks of the treatment. The levels of lindane in breast milk are 60 times higher than in untreated women, therefore this medication should be avoided during breastfeeding [32].

A unilateral rosacea-like chronic dermatitis in the right side of the face, which harbored innumerable *D. folliculorum* and *D. brevis*, was successfully treated with 10% crotamiton (Eurax) [33]. Forton et al. [34] analyzed the efficacy of six topical medications: metronidazole 2%, permethrin 1%, sublimed sulfur 10%, lindane 1%, crotamiton 10% and benzyl benzoate 10%. Their acaricidal activity was measured according to three criteria: (1) decrease of Demodex density to under the normal threshold; (2) significant decrease in Demodex density; and (3) comparison of the relative difference in Demodex density between treatments. Benzyl benzoate demonstrated the best therapeutic effect providing the highest score in all three categories. The efficacy of crotamiton was demonstrated by the second criterion, while some irritation was observed with benzyl benzoate and sulfur.

Forstinger et al. [35] reported the case of a patient with a chronic rosacea-like dermatitis of the facial skin and the eyelids, whose skin scrapings and a histological examination of a biopsy specimen from the affected area revealed the presence of numerous Demodex mites. The patient was treated with oral ivermectin 200 µg/kg (a macrocyclic lactone with broad-spectrum antiparasitic properties) and subsequent topical permethrin 5%, resulting in complete and rapid clearing of the folliculitis. Clyti et al. [36] reported the case of a patient infected by HIV and successfully treated with 2 doses of ivermectin with one month interval for disseminated demodicosis, presented with a pruritic eruption on the face as well as on the pre-sternal and interscapular areas. Allen et al. [37] successfully treated a case of papulopustular rosacea in an immunocompetent patient by oral ivermectin and topical 5% permethrin. A combination of ivermectin and permethrin for the treatment of demodicosis was also used earlier by Aquilina et al. [38], Damian & Rogers [39].

Our personal experience with ivermectin also signifies its great efficacy. However, high recurrence rates demonstrate an insufficiency of single dose administration. Several applications should be envisaged during ivermectin treatment. First of all, it should be given preferably in the evening, when the Demodex mites are leaving the pilosebacous areas in order to mate on the skin surface. Secondly, due to the fact that ivermectin does not have ovicidal properties, it is recommended to repeat the treatment two or three times, with intervals of 1 or 2 weeks (a plasmatic half-time of the drug after oral administration is 36 h). Thirdly, an intramuscular injection may be applied in non-compliant patients. Fourthly, additional acaricidal medications for topical application can not only provide some synergistic effect, but could also be useful in the maintenance of exposure to acaricides when ivermectin is metabolized and no longer active.

Kocak et al. [40] reported a study with 63 patients diagnosed as having papulopustular rosacea based on the clinical and histological findings. Patients were randomly assigned into 5% permethrin (n = 23), 0.75% metronidazole (n = 20) and placebo (n = 20) groups. Scores of erythema, telangiectasia, edema and rhinophyma and the number of papules, pustules, inflammatory nodules and *D. folliculorum* were determined. Applied twice daily the effect of permethrin on *D. folliculorum* was superior to that of metronidazole gel. The effect of permethrin cream on erythema and papules was found to be more effective than placebo and as effective as metronidazole gel. However, it had no effect on telangiectasia, rhinophyma and pustules. Xia et al. [41] treated 447 patients with Demodex infection on the face with a di-n-butyl phthalate-OP emulsion. Twenty days after treatment, the negative conversion rate and the therapeutic effect were evaluated and the authors came to the conclusion that the emulsion was significantly more effective than 2% and 8% metronidazole. Zang et al. [42] found that a 2% sodium dodecylbenzene sulfonate had a high in vitro killing effect on Demodex and was highly effective in the treatment of demodicosis.

Treatment of demodex blepharitis

Fulk & Clifford [43] reported on a patient who had an excessive number of *D. folliculorum* on his eyelashes. The primary symptom of itching was relieved after one week of treatment and the number of mites was reduced after 3 weeks of treatment with mercuric oxide ointment. Although being a strong acaricide, mercuric oxide ointment due to its systemic toxicity should be avoided.

Fulk et al. [44] evaluated 4% pilocarpine gel as a treatment for Demodex blepharitis. One eye was treated with pilocarpine gel, while the other eye remained untreated. The relative abundance of mites was evaluated at baseline, and after 1 and 2 weeks of treatment. In 11 out of 22 patients with ocular itching, the number of mites decreased significantly by the treatment, and the amount of mite reduction was closely correlated with the extent to which itching was alleviated. Our experience with pilocarpine gel showed that this medication works instantly and provides great relief for patients. However, the effect of pilocarpine is apparently rather acarostatic than acaricidal, providing a dose-dependent inhibition of the respiratory and nervous system. Because it is not ovicidal also in this case several treatments are required.

Demmler et al. [45] examined 3,152 cilia from 139 patients with blepharitis (38% blepharitis, 44% blepharo-conjunctivitis and 18% with other eye ailments) and 108 control individuals for Demodex. Demodex-positive blepharitis patients (n = 41) were treated for 3 weeks with mercury ointment (2%), lindane, cortisone or antibiotics. Of the patients with Demodex, 25% had no more parasites after mercury ointment or lindane creme, and 15% after cortisone and antibiotic treatments.

Rodriguez et al. [46] examined the eyelashes of 20 subjects with chronic blepharitis and 105 subjects without blepharitis. The incidence of Demodex infestation in the control group was 0.08 mites per eyelash, whereas in the patients with chronic blepharitis the incidence was 0.69 mites per eyelash. After 3-8 weeks of specific treatment the number of mites per eyelash in patients with chronic blepharitis decreased significantly, while 2 patients showed intolerance to the therapy.

Gao et al. [47] reported the clinical outcome of treating ocular demodicosis by lid scrub with 50% tea tree oil, which is known to be an effective pediculicide. Of eleven patients who were treated weekly, the Demodex count dropped to 0 for 2 consecutive visits in less than 4 weeks in 8 of 11 patients. Ten of the 11 patients showed different degrees of symptomatic relief and notable reduction of inflammatory signs. Significant visual improvement in 6 of 22 eyes was associated with a stable lipid tear film caused by significant reduction of lipid spread time, while lid scrub with tea tree oil caused notable irritation in 3 patients.

Conclusions

- It is of paramount importance to make the right diagnosis of Demodex mite infestation in relation to the main skin problem, as well as to establish Demodex as an etiological agent for blepharitis by finding large numbers of mites in the follicles and/or eyelashes, before a treatment with acaricides is initiated.
- In order to prevent a flare-up reaction of the entire face, which could appear after a treatment with acaricide such as lindane, it might be advisable to treat first a smaller segment of the infested area.
- A treatment should last for several weeks, even if the symptoms disappear earlier.
- More than two acaricides with overlapping mechanisms of action may be required for an effective treatment

References

1. Georgala S, Katoulis AC, Kylafis GD, Koumantaki-Mathioudaki E, Georgala C, Aroni K. Increased density of *Demodex folliculorum* and evidence of delayed hypersensitivity reaction in subjects with papulopustular rosacea. J Eur Acad Dermatol Venereol 2001; 15: 441-444.
2. el-Shazly AM, Ghaneum BM, Morsy TA, Aaty HE. The pathogenesis of *Demodex folliculorum* (hair follicular mites) in females with and without rosacea. J Egypt Soc Parasitol 2001; 31: 867-875.
3. Madeira NG, Sogayar MI. *Demodex folliculorum* e *Demodex brevis* em uma amostra da populacao de Botucatu, Sao Paulo, Brasil. Rev Soc Bras Med Trop 1993; 26: 221-224.
4. Akilov OE, Mumcuoglu KY. Association between human demodicosis and HLA class I. Clin Exp Dermatol 2003; 28: 70-73.
5. Kaufman-Wolf M. Concerning the usual presence of *Demodex folliculorum* in the pustules of acne rosacea. Derm Wschr 1925; 81: 1095-1103.
6. Ayres S. Pityriasis folliculorum (Demodex) Arch Derm Syph 1930; 21: 19-24.
7. Ayres S, Anderson NP. *Demodex folliculorum.* Arch Dermatol 1932; 25: 89.
8. Ayres S, Ayres S. Demodectic eruptions (demodicidosis) in the human. Arch. Dermatol. 1961; 83: 816-827.
9. Russell BF. Some aspects of the biology of the epidermis. BMJ 1962; i: 815-820.
10. Spickett SG. Aetiology of rosacea. BMJ 1962; i: 1625-1626.

11. Pallotta S, Cianchini G, Martelloni E, Ferranti G, Girardelli CR, Di Lella G, Puddu P. Unilateral demodicidosis. Eur J Dermatol 1998; 8: 191-192.

12. Franklin CD, Underwood JC. Demodex infestation of oral mucosal sebaceous glands. Oral Surg Oral Med Oral Pathol 1986; 61: 80-82.

13. Amichai B, Grunwald MH, Avinoach I, Halevy S. Granulomatous rosacea associated with *Demodex folliculorum*. Int J Dermatol 1992; 31: 718-719.

14. Basta-Juzbasic A, Marinovic T, Dobric I, Bolanca-Bumber S, Sencar J. The possible role of skin surface lipid in rosacea with epitheloid granulomas. Acta Med Croatica 1992; 46: 119-123.

15. Farina MC, Requena L, Sarasa JL, Martin L, Escalonilla P, Soriano ML, Grilli R, De Castro A. Spinulosis of the face as a manifestation of demodicidosis. Br J Dermatol 1998; 138: 901-903.

16. Grossmann B, Jung K, Linse R. [Tubero-pustular demodicosis]. Hautarzt 1999; 50: 491-494.

17. de Jaureguiberry JP, Carsuzaa F, Pierre C, Arnoux D, Jaubert D. [Demodex folliculitis: a cause of pruritus in human immunodeficiency virus infection]. Ann Med Interne (Paris) 1993; 144: 63-64.

18. Redondo Mateo J, Soto Guzman O, Fernandez Rubio E, Dominguez Franjo F. Demodex-attributed rosacea-like lesions in AIDS. Acta Derm Venereol 1993; 73: 437.

19. Barrio J, Lecona M, Hernanz JM, Sanchez M, Gurbindo MD, Lazaro P, Barrio JL. Rosacea-like demodicosis in an HIV-positive child. Dermatology 1996; 192: 143-145.

20. Aydingoz IE, Mansur T, Dervent B. Demodex folliculorum in renal transplant patients. Dermatology 1997; 195: 232-234.

21. Akbulatova L. [The pathogenic role of the mite Demodex and the clinical forms of demodicosis in man]. Vestn Dermatol Venerol 1966; 40: 57-61.

22. Akilov OE, Butov YS, Mumcuoglu KY. A clinico-pathological approach to the classification of human demodicosis. J German Soc Dermatol 2005; 3: 607-614.

23. Raehlmann E. Ueber Blepharitis acarica. Eine Erkrankung der Wimpern und Lidraender infolge von Milben in den Cilienbaelgen. Klin Mbl Augenheilk 1899; 37: 33.

24. Morgan RJ, Coston TO. Demodex blepharitis. Sth Med J Nashville 1964; 57: 694-699.

25. Ayres S, Mihan R. Rosacea-like demodicosis involving the eyelids. Archs Derm 1967; 95: 63-66.

26. Post C, Juhlin E. *Demodex folliculorum* and blepharitis. Archs Derm 1963; 88: 298-302.

27. Turk M, Ozturk I, Sener AG, Kucukbay S, Afsar I, Maden A. Comparison of incidence of *Demodex folliculorum* on the eyelash follicule in normal people and blepharitis patients. Turkiye Parazitol Derg 2007; 31: 296-297.

28. Czepita D, Kuźna-Grygiel W, Czepita M, Grobelny A. *Demodex folliculorum* and *Demodex brevis* as a cause of chronic marginal blepharitis. Ann Acad Med Stetin 2007; 53: 63-67.

29. Nutting WB, Green AC. Pathogenesis associated with hair follicle mites (*Demodex spp*) in Australian aborigines. Br J Derm 1976; 94: 307-312.

30. Desch C, Nutting WB. *Demodex folliculorum* (Simon) and *D. brevis* Akbulatova of man: redescription and reevaluation. J Parasit 1972; 58: 169-177.

31. Rufli T, Mumcuoglu Y, Cajacob A, Büchner S. [*Demodex folliculorum*: aetiopathogenesis and therapy of rosacea and perioral dermatitis] [in German]. Dermatologica 1981; 162: 12-26.

32. Ross TC, Alam M, Roos S, et al. Pharmacotherpay of ectoparastic infections, Drugs 2001: 61: 1067-1088.

33. Shelley WB, Shelley ED, Burmeister V. Unilateral demodectic rosacea. J Am Acad Dermatol 1989; 20: 915-917.

34. Forton F, Seys B, Marchal JL, Song AM. *Demodex folliculorum* and topical treatment: acaricidal action evaluated by standardized skin surface biopsy. Br J Dermatol 1998; 138: 461-466.

35. Forstinger C, Kittler H, Binder M. Treatment of rosacea-like demodicidosis with oral ivermectin and topical permethrin cream. J Am Acad Dermatol 1999; 41: 775-777.

36. Clyti E, Sayavong K, Chanthavisouk K. [Demodecidosis in a patient infected by HIV: successful treatment with ivermectin] [in French] Ann Dermatol Venereol 2005; 132: 459-461.

37. Allen KJ, Davis CL, Billings SD, Mousdicas N. Recalcitrant papulopustular rosacea in an immunocompetent patient responding to combination therapy with oral ivermectin and topical permethrin. Cutis. 2007; 80: 149-151.

38. Aquilina C, Viraben R, Sire S. Ivermectin-responsive Demodex infestation during human immunodeficiency virus infection. A case report and literature review. Dermatology 2002; 205: 394-397.

39. Damian D, Rogers M. Demodex infestation in a child with leukaemia: treatment with ivermectin and permethrin. Int J Dermatol 2003; 42: 724-726.

40. Kocak M, Yagli S, Vahapoglu G, Eksioglu M. Permethrin 5% cream versus metronidazole 0.75% gel for the treatment of papulopustular rosacea. A randomized double-blind placebo-controlled study. Dermatology 2002; 205: 265-270.

41. Xia H, Hu SF, Ma WJ, Ge JH. [Studies of di-n-butyl phthalate-OP emulsion in the treatment of demodicidosis] [in Chinese]. Zhongguo Ji Sheng Chong Xue Yu Ji Sheng Chong Bing Za Zhi. 2004; 22: 248-249.

42. Zang Y, Wu DJ, Song JB. [Experimental and clinical studies on the effect of sodium dodecylbenzene sulfonate in in vitro killing Demodex and in treating demodicidosis] [in Chinese]. Zhongguo Ji Sheng Chong Xue Yu Ji Sheng Chong Bing Za Zhi. 2005; 23: 221-224.

43. Fulk GW, Clifford C. A case report of demodicosis. J Am Optom Assoc 1990; 61: 637-639.

44. Fulk GW, Murphy B, Robins MD. Pilocarpine gel for the treatment of demodicosis - a case series. Optom Vis Sci 1996; 73: 742-745.

45. Demmler M, de Kaspar HM, Möhring C, Klauss V. [Blepharitis. *Demodex folliculorum*, associated pathogen spectrum and specific therapy] [in German]. Ophthalmologe 1997; 94: 191-196.

46. Rodríguez AE, Ferrer C, Alió JL. [Chronic blepharitis and Demodex] [in Spanish]. Arch Soc Esp Oftalmol 2005; 80: 635-642

47. Gao YY, Di Pascuale MA, Elizondo A, Tseng SC. Clinical treatment of ocular demodecosis by lid scrub with tea tree oil. Cornea. 2007; 26: 136-143.

A Molecular Link Between Rosacea and Gastrointestinal Disease

JOANNE WHITEHEAD, PH.D.

Victoria, British Columbia, Canada
joanne@irosacea.org

Rosacea is a common inflammatory condition of the facial skin of unknown etiology, which frequently occurs in combination with gastrointestinal disorders. Many dietary and hormonal factors are known to affect the severity of rosacea symptoms, several of which also modulate the activity of the enzyme intestinal alkaline phosphatase (IAP). The role of IAP in inhibiting an inflammatory response to intestinal bacteria suggests a mechanism by which intestinal pathologies may be linked to the skin inflammation characteristic of rosacea. Analysis of alkaline phosphatase activity is routinely performed on blood samples, and methods to quantify enzyme activity of the intestinal isoform specifically have been described. Correlations between IAP activity and rosacea symptoms in patients and controls can thus be screened by noninvasive and inexpensive means. If IAP activity is found to be low in rosacea patients, acute symptoms could be treated with oral IAP supplementation, and trials of IAP-activating medications currently used in gastrointestinal disease could be initiated in rosacea patients. More importantly, the safe and long-term control of rosacea could be undertaken by patients themselves through dietary modification to naturally increase IAP activity.

Rosacea and gastrointestinal disorders

Rosacea is an acneform condition localized to the central region of the face, characterized by redness, inflammation and excessive vascularization. Symptoms present in various combinations and degrees of severity, and often fluctuate between periods of exacerbation and remission. Rosacea appears most frequently in fair skinned adults of northern European ancestry, with an estimated prevalence of 16% in Caucasian women [1]. A high frequency of comorbidity with gastrointestinal disorders is seen in rosacea patients, but findings have not been consistent across different populations. Watson et al. described a cohort of rosacea patients with intestinal dysplasia including complete absence of microvilli, in association with malabsorption and celiac disease [2]. Reports in the literature also describe comorbidity with the inflammatory bowel disorders, ulcerative colitis and Crohn's disease [3,4]. Reducing digestive transit time has been shown to reduce rosacea severity [5].

A role for gastrointestinal flora in rosacea has been suspected for several reasons. A higher frequency of *Helicobacter pylori* infection is seen in rosacea patients than the general population [6–9], and *H. pylori* eradication can reduce rosacea symptoms [10,11]. Rosacea patients have a high incidence of small intestinal bacterial overgrowth, and eradication of overgrowth correlates with elimination or reduction of symptoms, while the same treatment is ineffective in rosacea patients without intestinal bacterial overgrowth [12]. In addition, rosacea is commonly treated with systemic antibiotics such as tetracycline or metronidazole, which modify intestinal flora [13], although symptoms frequently recur after cessation of treatment.

Despite a large body of evidence linking gastrointestinal disorders and bacterial flora with rosacea, no common underlying mechanism linking the two phenotypes has yet been described. Here I present a potential molecular mechanism connecting the two inflammatory pathologies.

The IAP hypothesis

The comorbidity of intestinal pathologies with rosacea, as well as the documented response of rosacea symptoms to a range of dietary and hormonal factors, as described below, makes the enzyme intestinal alkaline phosphatase (IAP) an attractive candidate as a central player in the etiology of rosacea. IAP is a membrane-bound enzyme expressed on the surface of the intestinal brush border, which serves to dephosphorylate and thus detoxify lipopolysaccharide (LPS or endotoxin) from the surface of Gram negative bacteria in the digestive tract. This action inhibits the inflammatory response, in order to promote tolerance to normal intestinal flora [14,15]. If not detoxified, LPS induces transcription of proinflammatory cytokines including tumour necrosis factor alpha (TNFa), which can act both locally in the gut and systemically [14]. Elevated levels of the cytokines TNFa and interleukin-1β (IL-1β) are seen in several inflammatory conditions of the digestive tract, including inflammatory bowel disease, irritable bowel syndrome and celiac disease [16]. The production of these cytokines may lead to further reinforcement of the inflammatory effect, as TNFa and IL-1 β have been shown to inhibit transcription of IAP, thus further stimulating the inappropriate immune response [16].

Crohn's disease and ulcerative colitis result from an inappropriate immune response to normal intestinal flora, which may be a feature shared with rosacea. Both Crohn's and colitis are correlated with reduced IAP expression, particularly in regions of inflamed tissue [17,18], and the pathology of these diseases has been proposed to be triggered by LPS. Indeed, administration of oral IAP tablets to colitis-induced rats leads to reduced production of TNFa and IL-1 β proinflammatory cytokines [18]. As the intestinal brush border is the site of IAP production, rosacea patients observed to have short or absent intestinal villi [2] would be expected to have greatly reduced expression of IAP. Other intestinal pathologies correlated with rosacea have been shown to result in low IAP activity. For example, studies of celiac disease have demonstrated that IAP activity is reduced in the intestinal mucosa in untreated patients as compared to controls, correlating with the degree of mucosal damage [19–22], and that IAP activity normalizes in response to treatment [23,24]. The use of systemic antibiotics for rosacea treatment may therefore act by reducing the load of LPS-carrying bacteria in the intestine, thus reducing both local and global inflammatory effects. Systemic metronidazole is often the first treatment option for rosacea, and is also commonly prescribed for inflammatory bowel disease and Crohn's disease. Indeed, metronidazole has been shown to elevate IAP activity [25] and reduce TNF levels [26].

Dietary modulation of IAP activity and rosacea

Much anecdotal knowledge is available on the role of diet in modifying rosacea symptoms [27,28], although identified dietary trigger factors vary between individuals. Due to the difficulties inherent in running sufficiently well controlled dietary intervention trials, no solid clinical evidence for an anti-rosacea diet has yet been presented.

The lack of consistency in identifying specific food triggers may be explained by considering that the metabolic effect of the diet as a whole could be more relevant than that of individual foods. The optimal pH for IAP activity in vitro is in the range of 9–10, but it has been shown to function effectively at the physiological pH of 7.5 in the intestine using LPS as a substrate [29]. Metabolic acidosis, caused by eating a typical modern western diet high in processed foods and low in fresh fruits and vegetables, giving a net renal acid load, is reflected in an acidic urine pH [30], likely reflecting a suboptimal pH for IAP enzymatic activity within the digestive tract. The striking effects of changing to an alkalizing diet on minimizing the inflammation of rosacea [31] [personal observations] may therefore be due to improved IAP activity.

In addition to the proposed role for the overall metabolic acid/ base balance on IAP, several dietary factors have been shown to specifically modulate IAP activity. The enzyme is inhibited by phytates [32] (found in grains and legumes) and by phenylalanine [33] (a component of several artificial sweeteners). Short-chain fatty acids such as butyrate, derived from the fermentation in the gut of dietary fibre or ingested directly from butter, increase IAP activity [34]. Dietary fish oil increases IAP activity in the intestinal brush border, gut lumen and serum, both through an increased transcriptional rate and through higher enzyme secretion from the intestinal surface into surfactant-like particles [35,36]. This secretory effect was shown to act via the hormone cholecystokinin which is released in response to oil feeding [37,38].

IAP is also activated by dietary zinc [33] and by vitamin A [39–41]. The first clinical trial of zinc sulfate supplementation in rosacea patients showed significant improvements in symptoms of the study group as compared to the placebo group [42]. The synthetic vitamin A analogs such as isotretinoin which are used to treat severe rosacea and other forms of acne have also been shown to increase IAP activity [43], and as such may represent an additional unrecognized mode of action of these compounds.

Hormonal modulation of IAP activity and rosacea

Hormonal status is known to affect the severity of rosacea symptoms. Anecdotal evidence suggests that inflammation is reduced during the estrogen phase and increased during the progesterone phase of the menstrual cycle, that estrogen-based contraceptive use can stabilize symptoms, and that inflammation can increase with pregnancy, during which time progesterone remains elevated [44–47]. Rosacea onset has been documented in response to a progesterone-releasing intrauterine contraceptive device [48], and the onset of a severe form of rosacea can coincide with pregnancy [49].

These hormonal variations in rosacea severity correlate well with documented effects of hormones on IAP activity. Ovariectomy, which eliminates endogenous estrogen production, decreases IAP activity, while supplemental estradiol reactivates IAP activity in ovariectomized rats [50]. IAP activity is repressed by the hormonal contraceptive medroxyprogesterone acetate, likely due to its antiestrogenic effects [51]. These data show activating effects of estrogens and inhibitory effects of progesterones on IAP activity, and are consistent with the observed effects on rosacea symptoms.

Evaluation of the hypothesis

Analysis of alkaline phosphatase activity from blood samples is already routinely carried out in medical laboratories, providing a quick, inexpensive and minimally invasive testing method. As at least four isoforms are present in serum, further analysis needs to be done to attribute enzyme activity specifically to the intestinal isoform, but straightforward methods to do this have been described, either by electrophoretic or chromatographic separation of the isoforms, or by measuring changes in enzyme activity in response to inhibitors acting differentially on the isoforms [52]. By testing IAP activity in a cohort of rosacea patients, and controlling for endogenous and exogenous hormonal status, baseline IAP activity levels can be compared between rosacea patients and control subjects.

Enteric coated oral IAP tablets have been shown to reduce the inflammatory response in the intestine of rats [18]. Using an informative cohort of patients and appropriately matched controls, oral IAP enzyme could be administered, and correlated with a standardized grading system of rosacea symptoms [53]. If effective in reducing or eliminating skin inflammation, several pharmaceutical, hormonal and dietary means of modulating endogenous IAP activity could then be tested for use in the practical and safe long-term elimination of rosacea.

Consequences of the hypothesis

IAP makes an attractive candidate as a central mediator of the inflammatory symptoms of rosacea, and validation of this hypothesis would have multiple positive implications: treatment of acute symptoms would be possible by oral enzyme supplementation, the long-term reduction or elimination of symptoms could be achieved by dietary modification or supplementation, and better informed use of hormonal medications could be implemented. In addition, a specific target would be available for developing new and effective means of pharmaceutical intervention.

Pharmaceutical interventions for rosacea

The use of oral IAP of bovine origin for the treatment of ulcerative colitis is currently being tested, with phase I and II clinical trials demonstrating both safety and effectiveness in reducing LPS-induced inflammation, and recombinant human IAP is now under development [54]. Given the proposed shared mode of action between colitis and rosacea, this should also be an effective intervention for rosacea. Other medications already in use for the treatment of Crohn's disease and ulcerative colitis, such as 5-ASA sulfate, also improve IAP activity [55], and could easily be evaluated in an off-label trial for control of rosacea symptoms.

The vitamin A analogs sometimes used in rosacea treatment have high toxicity and carry risk of serious complications, so their use is often contraindicated and must be very closely monitored [56]. However, by considering IAP as an important molecular target, it may be possible to screen analogs or develop new chemical variants which can optimize IAP activity while minimizing interference with other physiological pathways, thus improving safety and reducing side effects. The use of intestinal tissue culture slices has already been developed as an in vitro system for monitoring drug metabolism and response to inducers or inhibitors of IAP activity [57]. This creates an excellent tool for the preclinical screening of these and other pharmaceuticals for use in rosacea treatment.

Recognizing the hormonal effects on IAP activity will also lead to better informed use of hormonal medications, such as selecting combination pills containing estrogen, rather than using progesterone alone for contraception. Contraceptives with anti-progesterone activity currently under development may also prove useful for rosacea patients [58].

Dietary interventions for rosacea

Should IAP activity be shown to correlate with the inflammatory symptoms of rosacea, then effective and low risk interventions would be easily available to rosacea patients themselves. Despite the difficulty in accurately calculating the net acid/base balance of individual foods, while accounting for the varying bioavailability of each nutrient and effects of metabolic transformation [59,60], it has been demonstrated that the net endogenous acid production can be closely estimated using only the total protein and potassium content of food [61]. In this way, it can be shown that protein-rich meats and dairy products, and potassium-poor cereal grains are net acid-producing foods, while foods rich in a variety of potassium salts, such as fruits, vegetables and nuts, are net base-producing foods, with legumes effectively neutral. By favouring base-producing foods in the diet, it should be possible to provide conditions within the digestive tract for optimal IAP activity.

In addition to an alkalizing diet, specific foods providing key nutrients to promote IAP activity could be regularly consumed, such as oysters for zinc, orange vegetables for beta-carotene (pro-vitamin A), and cold water fish for fish oils. Similarly, foods high in known inhibitors of IAP activity, such as phytates and artificial sweeteners, could be reduced or avoided (see Table 1).

Regular consumption of probiotics, such as found in cultured dairy products or lactofermented foods and drinks, may be beneficial in reducing rosacea symptoms, perhaps by promoting the colonization of the intestinal tract with beneficial Gram-positive bacteria, thus minimizing the overgrowth of LPS-containing Gram-negative bacteria. Indeed, probiotics have proven beneficial in reducing the inflammation of irritable bowel syndrome, in limiting intestinal bacterial overgrowth, and in promoting a favourable ratio of anti-inflammatory to pro-inflammatory cytokines [62–64].

While dietary optimization would be the ideal natural and safe approach, in patients for whom dietary modification is not feasible, carefully titrated nutritional supplementation should also be effective in reducing rosacea symptoms. Ideally, the effects of each of the proposed dietary modifications would be specifically assessed for their relative benefit in reducing rosacea symptoms, but such an IAP-promoting diet can nevertheless be implemented immediately and safely by any rosacea patient, and further optimized on an individual level for efficacy.

Table 1 Dietary recommendations for promoting IAP activity.

Maximize consumption of IAP activators

Oysters	Uniquely high in zinc [65]
Pumpkin, sweet potato, carrots	Rich in beta-carotene [65]
Herring, mackerel, salmon, sardines	Good source of fish oils
Butter	Source of butyrate
Fiber	Forms butyrate on fermentation in gut
Fresh fruits and vegetables	Negative renal acid load [61]
Lactofermented foods and drinks	Probiotic Gram-positive bacteria

Minimize consumption of IAP inhibitors

Phytates	Minimize by proper soaking and cooking of grains and legumes
Artificial sweeteners	Source of phenylalanine
Hard and processed cheeses, processed meats	High renal acid load [61]

Conclusions

The possibility that low IAP activity contributes to the pathology of rosacea provides an easily testable hypothesis, followed by opportunities for the direct reduction of symptoms by enzyme supplementation, and the long-term control of this disorder by safe and inexpensive dietary modification. This not only enables clinical trials in rosacea patients of medications already in use for digestive disorders, but provides rationale for the further optimization of current high risk rosacea medications such as the retinoids, and identifies a pharmaceutical target for the development of new medications. All of these possibilities could be implemented directly, with the help of established preclinical tissue culture models systems and standardized clinical analysis methodology.

References

[1] National Rosacea Society. New studies show high incidence of rosacea, and possible new causes, <http://www.rosacea.org/rr/2007/summer/article_1. php>; 2007 [accessed 02.09].

[2] Watson WC, Paton E, Murray D. Small-Bowel disease in rosacea. Lancet 1965;1:47–50.

[3] Walton S, Sheth M, Wyatt EH. Rosacea and ulcerative colitis: a possible association. J Clin Gastroenterol 1990;12:513–5.

[4] Romiti R, Jansen T, Heldwein W, Plewig G. Rosacea fulminans in a patient with Crohn's disease: a case report and review of the literature. Acta Dermatol Venereol 2000;80:127–9.

[5] Kendall SN. Remission of rosacea induced by reduction of gut transit time. Clin Exp Dermatol 2004;29:297–9.

[6] Zandi S, Shamsadini S, Zahedi MJ, Hyatbaksh M. Helicobacter pylori and rosacea. East Mediterr Health J 2003;9:167–71.

[7] Diaz C, O'Callaghan CJ, Khan A, Ilchyshyn A. Rosacea: a cutaneous marker of Helicobacter pylori infection? Results of a pilot study. Acta Derm Venereol 2003;83:282–6.

[8] Argenziano G, Donnarumma G, Iovene MR, Arnese P, Baldassarre MA, Baroni A. Incidence of anti-Helicobacter pylori and anti-CagA antibodies in rosacea patients. Int J Dermatol 2003;42:601–4.

[9] Gurer MA, Erel A, Erbas D, Caglar K, Atahan C. The seroprevalence of Helicobacter pylori and nitric oxide in acne rosacea. Int J Dermatol 2002;41:768–70.

[10] Boixeda de Miquel D, Vazquez Romero M, Vazquez Sequeiros E, et al. Effect of Helicobacter pylori eradication therapy in rosacea patients. Rev Esp Enferm Dig 2006;98:501–9.

[11] Szlachcic A. The link between Helicobacter pylori infection and rosacea. J Eur Acad Dermatol Venereol 2002;16:328–33.

[12] Parodi A, Paolino S, Greco A, et al. Small intestinal bacterial overgrowth in rosacea: clinical effectiveness of its eradication. Clin Gastroenterol Hepatol 2008;6:759–64.

[13] Borglund E, Hagermark O, Nord CE. Impact of topical clindamycin and systemic tetracycline on the skin and colon microflora in patients with acne vulgaris. Scand J Infect Dis Suppl 1984;43:76–81.

[14] Bates JM, Akerlund J, Mittge E, Guillemin K. Intestinal alkaline phosphatase detoxifies lipopolysaccharide and prevents inflammation in zebrafish in response to the gut microbiota. Cell Host Microbe 2007;2:371–82.

[15] Goldberg RF, Austen Jr WG, Zhang X, et al. Intestinal alkaline phosphatase is a gut mucosal defense factor maintained by enteral nutrition. Proc Natl Acad Sci USA 2008;105:3551–6.

[16] Malo MS, Biswas S, Abedrapo MA, Yeh L, Chen A, Hodin RA. The proinflammatory cytokines, IL-1beta and TNF-alpha, inhibit intestinal alkaline phosphatase gene expression. DNA Cell Biol 2006;25:684–95.

[17] Arvanitakis C. Abnormalities of jejunal mucosal enzymes in ulcerative colitis and Crohn's disease. Digestion 1979;19:259–66.

[18] Tuin A, Poelstra K, Jager-Krikken AD, et al. Role of alkaline phosphatase in colitis in man and rats. Gut 2008.

[19] Prasad KK, Thapa BR, Nain CK, Sharma AK, Singh K. Brush border enzyme activities in relation to histological lesion in pediatric celiac disease. J Gastroenterol Hepatol 2008;23:e348–352.

[20] O'Grady JG, Stevens FM, Keane R, et al. Intestinal lactase, sucrase, and alkaline phosphatase in 373 patients with coeliac disease. J Clin Pathol 1984;37:298–301.

[21] Andersen KJ, Schjonsby H, Skagen DW, Haga HJ. Enzyme activities in jejunal biopsy samples from patients with adult coeliac disease with and without steatorrhoea. Scand J Gastroenterol 1983;18:365–8.

[22] Lehmann FG, Hillert U. Fecal intestinal alkaline phosphatase in coeliac disease. Z Gastroenterol 1980;18:381–8.

[23] Mitchison HC, al Mardini H, Gillespie S, Laker M, Zaitoun A, Record CO. A pilot study of fluticasone propionate in untreated coeliac disease. Gut 1991;32:260–5.

[24] Andersen KJ, Schjonsby H, Skagen DW. Jejunal mucosal enzymes in untreated and treated coeliac disease. Scand J Gastroenterol 1983;18:251–6.

[25] Sanyal SN, Jamba L, Channan M. Effect of the antiprotozoal agent metronidazole (Flagyl) on absorptive and digestive functions of the rat intestine. Ann Nutr Metab 1992;36:235–43.

[26] Colpaert S, Liu Z, De Greef B, Rutgeerts P, Ceuppens JL, Geboes K. Effects of antitumour necrosis factor, interleukin-10 and antibiotic therapy in the indometacin-induced bowel inflammation rat model. Aliment Pharmacol Ther 2001;15:1827–36.

[27] National Rosacea Society. Rosacea triggers, <http://www.rosacea.org/patients/materials/triggersindex.php>; 2008 [accessed 02.09].

[28] American Academy of Dermatology. Food and drink: tips for monitoring your diet, <http://www.skincarephysicians.com/rosaceanet/controlling_flareups.html#3>; 2008 [accessed 02.09].

[29] Poelstra K, Bakker WW, Klok PA, Kamps JA, Hardonk MJ, Meijer DK. Dephosphorylation of endotoxin by alkaline phosphatase in vivo. Am J Pathol 1997;151:1163–9.

[30] Welch AA, Mulligan A, Bingham SA, Khaw KT. Urine pH is an indicator of dietary acid-base load, fruit and vegetables and meat intakes: results from the European Prospective Investigation into Cancer and Nutrition (EPIC)-Norfolk population study. Br J Nutr 2008;99:1335–43.

[31] Rosacea-Ltd. The rosacea diet, <http://www.rosacea-ltd.com/rosaceadiet.php3>; 2008 [accessed 02.09].

[32] Bitar K, Reinhold JG. Phytase and alkaline phosphatase activities in intestinal mucosae of rat, chicken, calf, and man. Biochim Biophys Acta 1972;268:442–52.

[33] Blanchard RK, Cousins RJ. Regulation of intestinal gene expression by dietary zinc: induction of uroguanylin mRNA by zinc deficiency. J Nutr 2000;130: 1393S–8S.

[34] Meng S, Wu JT, Archer SY, Hodin RA. Short-chain fatty acids and thyroid hormone interact in regulating enterocyte gene transcription. Surgery 1999;126:293–8.

[35] Grewal R, Mahmood A. Coordinated secretion of alkaline phosphatase into serum and intestine in fat-fed rats. Indian J Gastroenterol 2004;23:175–7.

[36] Kaur J, Madan S, Hamid A, Singla A, Mahmood A. Intestinal alkaline phosphatase secretion in oil-fed rats. Dig Dis Sci 2007;52:665–70.

[37] Gotze H, Adelson JW, Hadorn HB, Portmann R, Troesch V. Hormone-elicited enzyme release by the small intestinal wall. Gut 1972;13:471–6.

[38] Eliakim R, Mahmood A, Alpers DH. Rat intestinal alkaline phosphatase secretion into lumen and serum is coordinately regulated. Biochim Biophys Acta 1991;1091:1–8.

[39] Nikawa T, Rokutan K, Nanba K, et al. Vitamin A up-regulates expression of bone-type alkaline phosphatase in rat small intestinal crypt cell line and fetal rat small intestine. J Nutr 1998;128:1869–77.

[40] Riley PA, Spearman RI. Vitamin A-induced synthesis of alkaline phosphatase. Science 1968;160:1006–7.

[41] Zaiger G, Nur T, Barshack I, Berkovich Z, Goldberg I, Reifen R. Vitamin A exerts its activity at the transcriptional level in the small intestine. Eur J Nutr 2004;43:259–66.

[42] Sharquie KE, Najim RA, Al-Salman HN. Oral zinc sulfate in the treatment of rosacea: a double-blind, placebo-controlled study. Int J Dermatol 2006;45:857–61.

[43] Marsden JR, Trinick TR, Laker MF, Shuster S. Effects of isotretinoin on serum lipids and lipoproteins, liver and thyroid function. Clin Chim Acta 1984;143:243–51.

[44] National Rosacea Society. Rosacea review, <http://www.rosacea.org/rr/2002/ summer/ article_3.php>; 2002 [accessed 02.09].

[45] Fitzgerald MA. Diagnosis and treatment of rosacea. Advanced Studies in Nursing 2005;3:234–8.

[46] Dermis.net. What causes rosacea? <http://rosacea.dermis.net/content/e01geninfo/ e02pathogenesis/index_eng.html>; 2009 [accessed 02.09].

[47] National Rosacea Society. Rosacea review, <http://www.rosacea.org/rr/2008/winter/ article_2.php>; 2008 [accessed 02.09].

[48] Choudry K, Humphreys F, Menage J. Rosacea in association with the progesterone-releasing intrauterine contraceptive device. Clin Exp Dermatol 2001;26:102.

[49] Ferahbas A, Utas S, Mistik S, Uksal U, Peker D. Rosacea fulminans in pregnancy: case report and review of the literature. Am J Clin Dermatol 2006;7:141–4.

[50] Singh R, Nagapaul JP, Majumdar S, Chakravarti RN, Dhall GI. Effects of 17 betaestradiol and progesterone on intestinal digestive and absorptive functions in ovariectomized rats. Biochem Int 1985;10:777–86.

[51] Nagpaul JP, Kaushal M, Majumdar S, Mahmood A. Effect of various doses of medroxyprogesterone acetate on intestinal functions in rats. Indian J Gastroenterol 1990;9:45–7.

[52] Tillyer CR, Rakhorst S, Colley CM. Multicomponent analysis for alkaline phosphatase isoenzyme determination by multiple linear regression. Clin Chem 1994;40:803–10.

[53] Wilkin J, Dahl M, Detmar M, et al. Standard grading system for rosacea: report of the National Rosacea Society Expert Committee on the classification and staging of rosacea. J Am Acad Dermatol 2004;50:907–12.

[54] AM_Pharma. Alkaline phosphatase for treatment of Ulcerative Colitis, <http://www.am-pharma.com/>; 2008 [accessed 02.09].

[55] Herzog R, Leuschner J. Experimental studies on the pharmacokinetics and toxicity of 5-aminosalicylic acid-O-sulfate following local and systemic application. Arzneimittelforschung 1995;45:300–3.

[56] Ellis CN, Krach KJ. Uses and complications of isotretinoin therapy. J Am Acad Dermatol 2001;45:S150–7.

[57] van de Kerkhof EG, De Graaf IA, De Jager MH, Groothuis GM. Induction of phase I and II drug metabolism in rat small intestine and colon in vitro. Drug Metab Dispos 2007;35:898–907.

[58] Van Look PF, von Hertzen H. Clinical uses of antiprogesterones. Hum Reprod Update 1995;1:19–34.

[59] Remer T. Influence of nutrition on acid-base balance–metabolic aspects. Eur J Nutr 2001;40:214–20.

[60] Remer T, Manz F. Potential renal acid load of foods and its influence on urine pH. J Am Diet Assoc 1995;95:791–7.

[61] Frassetto LA, Morris Jr RC, Sebastian A. A practical approach to the balance between acid production and renal acid excretion in humans. J Nephrol 2006;19(Suppl. 9):S33–40.

[62] Barrett JS, Canale KE, Gearry RB, Irving PM, Gibson PR. Probiotic effects on intestinal fermentation patterns in patients with irritable bowel syndrome. World J Gastroenterol 2008;14:5020–4.

[63] O'Mahony L, McCarthy J, Kelly P, et al. Lactobacillus and bifidobacterium in irritable bowel syndrome: symptom responses and relationship to cytokine profiles. Gastroenterology 2005;128:541–51.

[64] McCarthy J, O'Mahony L, O'Callaghan L, et al. Double blind, placebo controlled trial of two probiotic strains in interleukin 10 knockout mice and mechanistic link with cytokine balance. Gut 2003;52:975–80.

[65] USDA Nutrient Data Laboratory. National nutrient database for standard reference, <http://www.nal.usda.gov/fnic/foodcomp/search/>; 2008 [accessed 02.09].

Reprinted from Medical Hypotheses 2009, 73(6):1019-1022, Whitehead J. Intestinal alkaline phosphatase: The molecular link between rosacea and gastrointestinal disease?
DOI: 10.1016/j.mehy.2009.02.049 Copyright 2009, with permission from Elsevier.

Signal Transduction Modulators to Treat Rosacea

Jeffry B. Stock, Ph.D.

Signum Biosciences, Monmouth Junction, New Jersey, USA
Department of Molecular Biology, Princeton University, Princeton, New Jersey, USA
www.signumbiosciences.com
jstock@signumbio.com
jstock@princeton.edu

Although rosacea is a common chronic inflammatory condition affecting over 14 million people nationwide every year (FoxAnalytics 2007; Crandall 2008), the etiology and pathology of this disease remain poorly understood. There is general agreement that rosacea is primarily an inflammatory disease, possibly associated with microbial and stress-related triggers. This view is supported by histopathologic findings that include follicular and perivascular leukocytic infiltrates (Feldman, Hollar et al. 2001; Powell 2005; Lacey, Delaney et al. 2007). It is further reinforced by research demonstrating that the antibiotics effective against rosacea work by suppressing a variety of proinflammatory mediators thought to play a primary role in rosacea pathophysiology (Dahl 2001; Korting and Schollmann 2009). Whereas topical agents, such as Metrogel®, Clindamycin, Clindamycin-Benzoyl peroxide, Sodium Sulfacetamide / Sulfur and Finacea® exhibit beneficial effects for the treatment of papulopustular (Type 2) rosacea, they tend to be less effective for the treatment of erythematotelangiectatic (Type 1) rosacea.

At Signum Biosciences, we are developing a novel class of topical Signal Transduction Modulators (STMs) that target several stages of the inflammatory cascade, resulting in a significant reduction of redness and erythema. This class of anti-inflammatory STMs inhibits inflammation by reducing the release of critical inflammatory mediators that underlie rosacea pathogenesis, including tumor necrosis factor alpha, interleukins IL-1, IL-6, and IL-8. This leads to a dramatic reduction in neutrophil infiltration and the consequent production of toxic reactive oxygen species.

STMs work by targeting regulatory enzymes that function to generate inflammation in the skin. These signaling components are termed G-proteins (Figure 1). Each G-protein contains a characteristic chemical group termed a polyisoprenoid tail that functions to target the G-protein to a polyisoprenoid-binding "pocket" that facilitates binding and proper signaling (Kloog and Cox 2004). STMs are structural mimics of this tail so they compete with G-protein binding so as to inhibit signaling and thereby block inflammation (Figure 1).

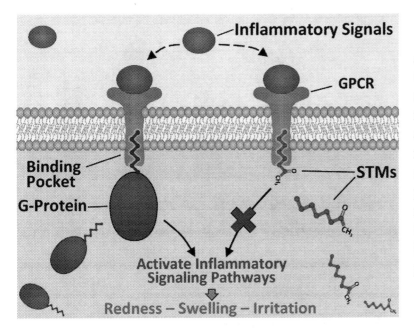

***Figure 1*. STMs modulate G-protein inflammatory signaling.** Through their novel mechanism of action, STMs successfully modulate inflammatory signaling by binding to prenyl-binding pockets, normally used by G-proteins to activate inflammation signaling pathways.

Anti-inflammatory STMs, also called isoprenylcysteine analogs, were initially discovered by Dr. Jeffry B. Stock (co-founder of Signum Biosciences) in the course of an investigation of the chemistry that regulates the targeting of intracellular signal transduction G-proteins such as Ras, Rho, Rac, and Gγ (Volker, Lane et al. 1991; Volker, Pillinger et al. 1995). The archetype of this class is Arazine™ (*N*-acetyl-*S*-farnesylcysteine). Arazine™ and its derivatives have been shown to inhibit a wide range of different inflammatory responses both *in vitro* and *in vivo* (Volker, Lane et al. 1991; Huzoor-Akbar, Wang et al. 1993; Philips, Pillinger et al. 1993; Volker, Pillinger et al. 1995; Gordon, Wolanin et al. 2008).

To evaluate the efficacy of STMs as anti-inflammatories *in vivo*, a chemically-induced inflammatory model was utilized (Figure 2). The mouse ear model has been previously used to test whether topically applied anti-inflammatories inhibit the development of acute, chemically-induced dermal irritation (Van Arman 1974; Young, Wagner et al. 1983; De Young, Kheifets et al. 1989; Kotyuk, Raychaudhuri et al. 1993; Rao, Currie et al. 1993; Tramposch 1999) and to compare the members of differing classes of anti-inflammatory agents with multiple mechanisms of action (Tramposch 1999). Inflammatory endpoints typically used are reduction of redness and erythema, swelling and edema and neutrophil infiltration. Results were compared to pharmaceutical agents that are currently in use for the topical treatment of rosacea: metronidazole (Metrogel®), azelaic acid (Finacea®), and brimonidine (a potent vasoconstrictor). In this model system, the STMs that were tested generally had superior activity in reducing erythema (Figure 2). Topical agents currently available on the market (Finacea® and Metrogel®) offer 16% and 23% erythema inhibition in the assay, respectively, whereas STM compounds (SIG0990, SIG1189, SIG1209, SIG1192) show a much greater anti-inflammatory activity with inhibitory values ranging from 66% for SIG1189 to 71% for SIG0990.

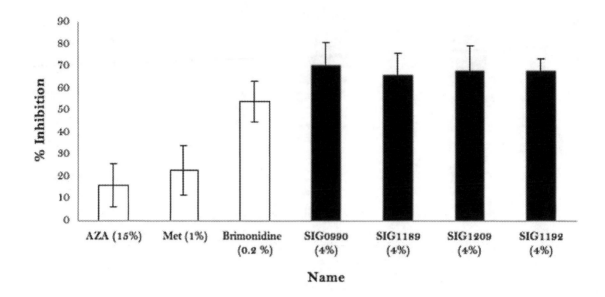

Figure 2. **Activity of STMs and topical rosacea treatments.** Using a mouse ear model of inflammation, compounds were tested for activity measuring for the reduction of erythema. Compounds azelaic acid (AZA/Finacea®), metronidazole (Metrogel®), brimonidine, STMs (SIG0990, SIG1189, SIG1209, SIG1192) were tested at the concentration shown.

In addition to their exceptional efficacy in reducing erythema, several potent STMs have now been synthesized that demonstrate strong activity in reducing neutrophil infiltration and edema, as well as blocking cytokine signaling (data not shown). Moreover, many of these agents also exhibit substantial anti-microbial activity that may enhance their utility for the treatment of rosacea. Besides their specific utility for the treatment of redness and rosacea, STMs represent a novel class of anti-inflammatories with strong therapeutic potential for several other inflammatory conditions such as acne, psoriasis, and atopic dermatitis. The first STM-based topical containing Arazine™ will be released to the Japanese market early in 2010.

References

Crandall, M. A. (2008). The Worldwide Market for Prescription Dermatological Drugs. Market Intelligence Report. K. Information. New York: 359.

Dahl, M. V. (2001). "Pathogenesis of rosacea." Advances in Dermatology **17**: 29-45.

De Young, L. M., J. B. Kheifets, et al. (1989). "Edema and cell infiltration in the phorbol ester-treated mouse ear are temporally separate and can be differentially modulated by pharmacologic agents." Agents and Actions **26**(3-4): 335-341.

Feldman, S. R., C. B. Hollar, et al. (2001). "Women commonly seek care for rosacea: dermatologists frequently provide the care." Cutis **68**(2): 156-160.

FoxAnalytics (2007). The Dermatology Market Outlook to 2011. B. I. LTD. London, UK: 201.

Gordon, J. S., P. M. Wolanin, et al. (2008). "Topical N-acetyl-S-farnesyl-L-cysteine inhibits mouse skin inflammation, and unlike dexamethasone, its effects are restricted to the application site." Journal of Investigative Dermatology **128**(3): 643-654.

Huzoor-Akbar, W. Wang, et al. (1993). "Protein prenylcysteine analog inhibits agonist-receptor-mediated signal transduction in human platelets." Proceedings of the National Academy of Sciences of the United States of America **90**(3): 868-872.

Kloog, Y. and A. D. Cox (2004). "Prenyl-binding domains: potential targets for Ras inhibitors and anti-cancer drugs." Seminars in Cancer Biology **14**(4): 253-261.

Korting, H. C. and C. Schollmann (2009). "Tetracycline Actions Relevant to Rosacea Treatment." Skin Pharmacol Physiol **22**(6): 287-294.

Kotyuk, B., A. Raychaudhuri, et al. (1993). "Effect of anti-inflammatory compounds on edema formation and myeloperoxidase activity in the arachidonic acid-induced ear model in the mouse." Agents and Actions **39 Spec No**: C46-48.

Lacey, N., S. Delaney, et al. (2007). "Mite-related bacterial antigens stimulate inflammatory cells in rosacea." Br J Dermatol **157**(3): 474-481.

Philips, M. R., M. H. Pillinger, et al. (1993). "Carboxyl methylation of Ras-related proteins during signal transduction in neutrophils." Science **259**(5097): 977-980.

Powell, F. C. (2005). "Clinical practice. Rosacea." New England Journal of Medicine **352**(8): 793-803.

Rao, T. S., J. L. Currie, et al. (1993). "Comparative evaluation of arachidonic acid (AA)- and tetradecanoylphorbol acetate (TPA)-induced dermal inflammation." Inflammation **17**(6): 723-741.

Tramposch, K. M. (1999). Skin Inflamation. *In Vivo* Models of Inflammation. D. W. Morgan and L. A. Marshall. Basel, Birkhäuser Verlag: 179-204.

Van Arman, C. G. (1974). "Anti-inflammatory drugs." Clinical Pharmacology and Therapeutics **16**(5 Part 2): 900-904.

Volker, C., P. Lane, et al. (1991). "A single activity carboxyl methylates both farnesyl and geranylgeranyl cysteine residues." FEBS Letters **295**(1-3): 189-194.

Volker, C., M. H. Pillinger, et al. (1995). "Prenylcysteine analogs to study function of carboxylmethylation in signal transduction." Methods in Enzymology **250**: 216-225.

Young, J. M., B. M. Wagner, et al. (1983). "Tachyphylaxis in 12-0-tetradecanoylphorbol acetate- and arachidonic acid-induced ear edema." Journal of Investigative Dermatology **80**(1): 48-52.

This work was presented at the Society for Investigative Dermatology meeting in Montreal, 2009 (poster 126):
"Isoprenylcysteine (IPC) analogs: a novel class of NSAIDs show activity to different inflammatory endpoints including reduced erythema".
E. Perez, J. B. Stock, A. V. Gonzalez, K. Rouzard, S.Y. Lee, M.V. Voronkov, K. Rapole,
J. Barrero-Oro, J. S. Gordon, M. B. Stock
Volume 129 supplement 1 April 2009. Supplement to the Journal of Investigative Dermatology

The Effect of Dietary Salt on Rosacea

Helen Cooper

RRDi Corporate Member
helen@irosacea.org

I don't know exactly when I went on a low-salt diet but it was many years ago. Too much salt was known to be a health risk and I reduced my intake. I had no problems until the spring of 2000 when I noticed that at meals I would take only a few bites and feel completely stuffed. Within a week red spots appeared on my nose and it wasn't long before I had full blown rosacea. I had been on a more extreme diet (vegetarian) for the two months prior, and suspected that there might be a connection. I immediately went back to eating my old favorites like burgers, fries, and ice cream. The rosacea improved but didn't go away. Every evening after supper I would have that bright red nose.

I made an appointment with my doctor who informed me that rosacea has absolutely nothing to do with diet and that there was no cure. In fact it was likely to get worse. She did prescribe Metrocreme®, but after a few weeks of use I found it to be of no benefit. Since this ailment did begin while I was on a diet, I wondered if my doctor could be wrong. I wondered what could be causing my face to flush, most noticeably after meals. I just knew my diet was the key to the riddle, but how? Was I getting too much or too little of something? Was it some kind of allergy? I had yet to make the low-salt / rosacea connection but began searching for information on the web.

The fact that I found most interesting was that hypochlorhydria (lack of stomach acid) is often present in rosaceans. In continuing my web search, this time looking for information on hypochlorhydria, I found a few sites indicating that salt is necessary for the body to manufacture stomach acid. Was it possible that rosacea is nothing but a salt deficiency? I hardly believed that a cure could be so simple, but I had nothing to lose so I began a diet higher in salt. Nothing changed for a quite a while but by the fourth month the flushing had subsided greatly. Over the next year or so it disappeared completely.

I was able to go back to being my normal self, but my faith in drugs, doctors and research was diminished. I had many questions. There have been so many amazing medical advances, why had this never been discovered? Was my experience simply an aberration? Why wasn't anyone with rosacea willing try my remedy or even discuss it? With one in 20 having this ailment, why have most people never heard of it? There are medications and cosmetics for rosacea but in searching the web I began reading about laser treatments and surgeries. Why had doctors never suggested any of these procedures and why did they show so little interest when it became apparent that I was cured? Was there no serious interest in finding a cure? My goal was to find answers to these questions and also come up with a theory as to why this high-salt diet caused a complete disappearance of all symptoms. The following is the theory I developed after my experiment with a salty diet.

Hydrochloric acid (HCl) is necessary for the digestion of food, and the chlorine molecule in salt (NaCl) is necessary for the stomach to manufacture this acid. The chlorine our body needs is found mainly in the salt we eat; however, low salt diets have become very popular and such a diet may be causing a salt deficiency. This salt deficiency, if severe enough, will result in a condition called hypochlorhydria (lack of stomach acid) and food will not digest properly. The body reacts by flushing blood, which contains salt, into the blood vessels surrounding the stomach to provide the chlorine necessary to create HCl. The digestive system, however, acts as a single unit and blood flushes into all parts of this system, not just the stomach. The nose and face are part of this digestive system and blood is continually flushing into this area as well. This flushing continues for weeks and months, and those of us who have a genetic tendency to blush are likely to develop this ailment. We have stretchy, delicate veins and capillaries, and chronic flushing causes these vessels to become enlarged and damaged, a condition we have named rosacea.

As to why my salt cure had never been discovered, the most alarming idea is that perhaps it has -- but remains unrevealed. There are products on the market that treat rosacea with varying degrees of success and keeping this salt cure a secret would protect profits. This brings up the interesting question as to whether or not a corporation has the responsibility to reveal its own medical discoveries. Is it legal to withhold information that would negatively impact a product already on the market? Could it be that the profit motive, which works so well in most areas of the economy, may have become a roadblock in the search for better cures?

I doubt, however, that there is a collusion to hide valuable information. It's just that the solution cannot be found in the laboratory. One could look at the entire planet and its population as another kind of lab, with billions of people living in different countries and being exposed to different diets and environments where cures could be discovered, perhaps accidentally. Unfortunately such things may never come to light -- because there's no one to tell. Even the greatest idea in the world needs a good salesman and a way to spread the news. With every business entity on the planet using the media to try to sell something, the public is bombarded. Publicizing a discovery is expensive and an insurmountable obstacle for the average person; it's easier to simply forget it and get on with life.

Medical professionals may not be very interested in rosacea because it is not considered a serious disease and recommending surgery or laser treatments might seem like hitting a fly with a sledgehammer. They know it to be incurable and may downplay it because there is no effective treatment for this ailment, the cause of which has been unknown for centuries. Consider that salt was rare until about 100 years ago, which would explain rosacea's persistence over the ages. Salt was used for currency at one time and was also considered to be a medicine but has gotten a bad rap in the last few decades. My theory is being ignored, not only because I am not a medical professional, but because the idea that common salt could cure anything sounds laughable.

The disease is not well known because of the embarrassment and shame associated with it. Some comments I received were, "Did you drink your lunch?" "Why is your nose so red?" The "fact" that it is an incurable "disease" that could cause deformities and loss of eyesight, is just too much to deal with. Feeling hopeless and in denial, we try various remedies, cover it with makeup, try not to think about it or talk about it and just hope it doesn't get much worse. Arthritis, injuries, allergies and many other ailments are open for discussion and an exchange of ideas. But there will be no rumors or grapevine remedies for rosacea. We don't want to embarrass anyone by mentioning it; this common ailment is a forbidden topic and has remained somewhat of a secret.

I suppose it is possible that my case is an aberration but emails I have received would suggest otherwise. Some replies to my salt theory were: "I can't eat much salt, it makes me puffy." "You may have something there, I went to a high-salt diet to increase my blood pressure and the rosacea got better." "I can't eat salt, I have high blood pressure." Some were resistant to the idea, eager to disagree and I wondered if they were on low-salt diets they did not want to give up.

Solving the puzzle, however, does not solve the problem. Many have discovered that dietary salt has the property of retaining water, causing weight gain. Low-salt diets are being used for the purpose of weight loss and it may be that nothing else has worked as well. Perhaps no one wants this "cure" and would rather be thinner and keep the rosacea! Fear of rosacea and its effects, however, could be a motivating factor in keeping off unwanted pounds, even though it means returning to more difficult diets. Our best hope may be that science will find better and better solutions to this problem of how to keep our weight within a normal range. Perhaps then we can put the salt shaker back on the table.

Is it Possible for Rosaceans to Do Research?

JOEL T. BAMFORD, M.D., F.A.A.D.

The Duluth Clinic, Duluth, Minnesota, USA
joeltm@irosacea.org

Take one simple question; only for example, "Are there common signs (visible changes) of rosacea, which are not on the face, extra facial in location?"

No single visible sign or lesion discussed here is diagnostic for rosacea. Diagnosis of rosacea depends on a combination of more than on type of sign and symptoms present. Usually a diagnosis is based on the presence of the classic redness, flushing, papules, pustules and telangiectasia on the face, or from eye findings. Evaluating an individual's concern, physicians look for each sign (erythema, scaling, telangiectasia, papules, pustules and edema) and each symptom present and review the history for migraine headache, and sties or dry eye symptoms such as burning or stinging. All of these have been statistically associated with rosacea. No single sign or symptom is enough to diagnose rosacea.

Two clinical studies have shown how skin changes associated with rosacea are very frequent on extra facial sites in rosaceans (Henderson 1995; Bamford 2002). In each study, using the same method, these changes (erythema, scaling, telangiectasia, papules, pustules and edema) were very similar. Specifically in Bamford et al, 42% - 84% have them. (For interest only, this study found that the lesions caused few symptoms). Rosaceans themselves, according to a National Rosacea Society member survey, reported that 25% were aware of extra facial rosacea.

Although the mentioned studies are published as posters, reviewers and editors have not wanted to publish these results until a case matched controlled study (rosaceans vs. randomly selected subjects without rosacea) is funded and completed. It would make an excellent subject for RRDi supported study, but done through standard dermatology office visits, it would be expensive. If it could be devised with volunteer effort (experts, planning, subjects, data assembly and writing), I believe it could lead to medical studies and information gathering and processing in a new, less costly direction.

It is a stretch to consider research by the people, as well as for the people; however, it is an important effort in this new environment of cutbacks in research funding.

References

Henderson CA, Charles-Holmes S, McSween R, Ilchyshyn A. A system for grading rosacea severity. Brit J Dermatol July 1995 (suppl).

Bamford, J., B. Elliott, et al. (2002). "The Relationship of Rosacea Phenotypes and Extra facial Lesions." (Poster 205) Society for Investigative Dermatology 119(1): 242 July 2002.

2009 Research Highlights

JOANNE WHITEHEAD, PH.D.

Editor in Chief
joanne@irosacea.org

In 2002, the National Rosacea Society Expert Committee on the Classification and Staging of Rosacea published a standard reference guide for classifying rosacea signs into four basic subtypes [1]. This was followed in 2004 by a standard grading system for assessing the severity of symptoms [2]. In 2009 the Expert Committee has released two papers in the journal *Cutis* describing an overview of rosacea care and recommended treatment modalities specific to each rosacea subtype and grade [3, 4]. Collectively, these important papers provide a common terminology for the discussion of rosacea, which facilitates diagnosis, management, and research.

A survey of members of the National Rosacea Society was carried out in 2006, with results reported in 2009 by Boni Elewski in the *Journal of Drugs in Dermatology* [5]. This survey gives a patients' perspective on how rosacea is addressed by doctors in the USA. While the survey did not provide direct data on the cure or remission of rosacea, 80 percent of respondents did report that medications stopped their symptoms from worsening, and more than one third of the 28 percent who took time off from their drug treatments did so due to relief of symptoms.

An important aspect of the survey was to assess whether patients were given adequate information by their health care providers, and many felt that discussion was lacking regarding adjunctive skin care, medication options, surgical or laser treatments, triggers, and physical or psychological symptoms. Although the study suffers from selection bias, in that the survey population was derived from patients actively seeking additional information on the internet, this does suggest that a subset of doctors treating rosacea lack either the time or the resources to discuss the condition in sufficient detail.

Due to the chronic nature of rosacea and the high rate of noncompliance with prescribed treatments, it is suggested that doctors stress the need for continuous drug therapy, even when symptoms disappear. However, it would be interesting, especially given the survey results, to compare this typical pharmacological approach to rosacea care with a more holistic model, in which drugs are used to manage acute phases of the disease, but adjunct skin care, trigger avoidance and lifestyle modifications are emphasized for the long term maintenance of skin health.

Writing in the *Journal of Cosmetic Dermatology*, Uwe Wollina and Shyam B. Verma propose that rosacea is more prevalent in India than previously recognized, so rather than being "the curse of the Celts", a disease specific to people of northern European ancestry, rosacea may have a wider distribution, consistent with the flow of people and their genes between

Europe and India early in human evolution [6]. By looking for chromosomal segments of European origin in Indian rosacea patients, researchers could now take advantage of this observation in narrowing down the search for potential genes determining predisposition to rosacea.

A comprehensive review of the molecular pathology of rosacea was published in the *Journal of Dermatological Science* in 2009 [7]. Based on their recent observation that rosacea patients show high levels of the antimicrobial peptide cathelicidin, which has both vasoactive and proinflammatory effects [8], Kenshi Yamasaki and Richard L. Gallo are able to unite different aspects of rosacea pathology through the perspective of innate immunity. Factors such as UV radiation, tissue damage and microbes including *Demodoex* mites and *Helicobacter pylori*, act on a hypersensitized innate immune system to induce the vascular changes and inflammation characteristic of rosacea. This unifying view of the various aspects of rosacea should prove to be a significant step forward in learning how to manage this disease.

References

[1]   Wilkin J, Dahl M, Detmar M, et al., Standard classification of rosacea: Report of the National Rosacea Society Expert Committee on the Classification and Staging of Rosacea. *J Am Acad Dermatol* **46** (2002), 584-587.

[2]   Wilkin J, Dahl M, Detmar M, et al., Standard grading system for rosacea: report of the National Rosacea Society Expert Committee on the classification and staging of rosacea. *J Am Acad Dermatol* **50** (2004), 907-912.

[3]   Odom R, Dahl M, Dover J, et al., Standard management options for rosacea, part 1: overview and broad spectrum of care. *Cutis* **84** (2009), 43-47.

[4]   Odom R, Dahl M, Dover J, et al., Standard management options for rosacea, part 2: options according to subtype. *Cutis* **84** (2009), 97-104.

[5]   Elewski BE, Results of a national rosacea patient survey: common issues that concern rosacea sufferers. *J Drugs Dermatol* **8** (2009), 120-123.

[6]   Wollina U and Verma SB, Rosacea and rhinophyma: not curse of the Celts but Indo Eurasians. *J Cosmet Dermatol* **8** (2009), 234-235.

[7]   Yamasaki K and Gallo RL, The molecular pathology of rosacea. *J Dermatol Sci* **55** (2009), 77-81.

[8]   Yamasaki K, Di Nardo A, Bardan A, et al., Increased serine protease activity and cathelicidin promotes skin inflammation in rosacea. *Nat Med* **13** (2007), 975-980.

Books to be Published in the Future

PROFESSOR GERD PLEWIG, M.D.

Department of Dermatology
Ludwig-Maximilian-University
Frauenlobstrasse 9-11
80337 Munich, Germany
gerd.plewig@med.uni-muenchen.de

Braun-Falco´s Dermatology. 3rd English edition. Walter Burgdorf, Gerd Plewig, Helmut Wolff and Michael Landthaler (editors). Springer-Verlag Heidelberg 2009. 1712 pages with 1200 colored figures. Includes Acne and Rosacea, chapter 67, pp 993-1017 by Gerd Plewig.

Pantheon der Dermatologie. Herausragende historische Persönlichkeiten « Pantheon of the Dermatology. Outstanding historical personalities » Christoph Löser and Gerd Plewig. Springer-Verlag Heidelberg 2008. 1186 pages and 1872 mostly colored figures. German. Includes notations of acne and rosacea.

Acne and Rosacea, 4th English edition, Springer-Verlag, Heidelberg. Gerd Plewig, Albert M. Kligman, Bodo Melnik and Thomas Jansen, to appear in 2010. 3rd edition included 744 pages with 216 colored plates.

74

Index